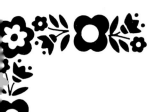

Contents

Foreword

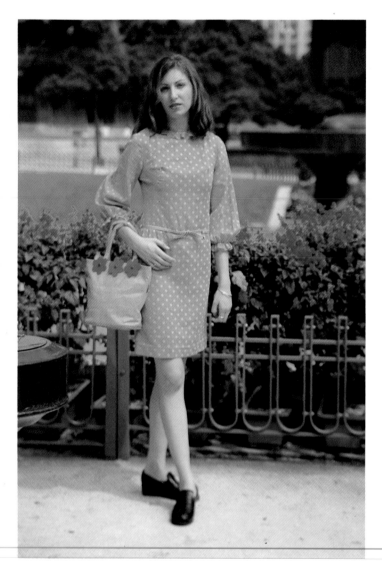

Lime green voile shift with hot pink polka dots and matching pink grosgrain ribbon belt. The only part of the label still left says it's 65% Dacron, so we can assume the other 35% is cotton. The orange handbag is from 1996.

Trina Robbins, whom I have known and admired since the 1970s, knows her gurus and groovy's, pill-boxes and platforms, patches and patchouli, paisley and peace-goods, hippie denims and hullabaloo Hawaiians, A-lines and Beene designs, bulging daisies and effulgent day-glow, polyester and Pop. In her fascinating guide to the days, nights, wrap skirts, and velvet blazers of the go-go years, Trina knows not only the clothes, but the culture of the 1960 and 1970s.

She gives us a fascinating history that is not only about fine ladies and best gear, but the full wardrobe of modern life. Trina knows how to track down not only the impressive labels of Pucci and Courreges, but the even more awe-inspiring white vinyl go-go boots, the unforgettable double-knit pantsuits, or the perky floral Lillies (Pulitzer, that is) that abounded in the time and now are the incredible discoveries of relentless searching and keen connoisseurship in second-hand shops and flea-marketing.

Trina mingles the perennials of the 1960s and 1970s with the fads. As she rightly recalls, those incredible velvet blazers — aping fin-de-siecle artists and aesthetes—brought Oscar Wilde to "The Partridge Family" and maxi-coats from *Doctor Zhivago* (look for Seventh-Avenue coat-manufacturer Abe Schrader's "Caviar Collection") became, for a slippery season, slush-catchers in New York City streets.

Too often, fashion is only about the most extravagant or about the most popular. Trina has chosen to focus on a time when popular and fabulous were synonymous and to help us discover equally the early Geoffrey Beene designs, recognize a denim-does-disco skirt, or savor the best of the incense-reeking boutiques entered through swinging bead curtains. Twiggy, in her 1968 autobiography, commented, "I've met a lot of rich people in the last year. And most of them are rich unhappy people. ... having money didn't make them have any fun." Trina, who personifies fantastic fashion, knows that crucial 1960-70s message. Fashion became something other than and better than the privilege of the rich. For Tiger Morse, for Twiggy, even girls in minis and micro-minis, for vinyl vixens, and gauzy, grannified little girls — half-Heidi, half-Mother-India — fashion wasn't about being rich or imitating the rich, it was about having fun.

Of course, there was Carnaby Street and Kings Road fun which still smacked of high style, but with Biba and collarless-jackets and Beatle-boots, there was the energy of rock and popular music. In both England and America, rock constituted a new energy and a new democracy for fashion: sometimes tailored like the early Beatles, sometimes pastiched and thrift-shop like the later (*Sgt. Pepper*, 1967) Beatles, sometimes

Rolling Stone scruffy, and sometimes Janis Joplin, Jimi Hendrix, and Roger Daltry native and dragging with the biggest and best fringe since the Charleston-dancing 1920s. Even the materials were fun: from the real leathers of rage and Black Panthers through the creaseless Dacron® and sponge-cleanable vinyl and psychedelic colors of 1967-68 paper dresses, a triumph of cheap chic. Diana Vreeland's bold *Vogue* years proclaimed that artificial materials was always better, brighter, and more theatrical than the real thing.

It was a mod, mod, mad, mad whirl and world. Airlines hired designers to make hip new uniforms for stewardesses. Skirts dematerialized and colorful stockings declared a new tribe. Jeans percolated from protest and populism into mainstream fashion. Political-resistance style often fast became disco duds. And that ubiquitous happy face smiled throughout.

You'll smile, too, throughout Trina's book. It is a marvelous cache of information and a hoard of memories (or for the younger set, historical items). It is a great, indispensable guide for collecting fashion's best in the era when fashion was at its best and most exuberant. If you want to remember when Joey Dee replaced Sandra Dee, if you want to recall when Chubby Checker was a lot more fun than playing checkers, and you want to know how to strike gold in a big polka-dotted miniskirt for doing the Watusi, this is the book for you.

"In the Sixties," wrote Marylin Bender in *The Beautiful People* (1967), "fashion stopped being clothes and became a value, a tool, a way of life, a kind of symbolism." Trina knows that, but she also knows that you can still, following her brilliant, colorful manual, find vintage clothes that defined the values and made THE SYMBOLS and, most important of all, produced THE FUN. Historians will, one day, tell us all about the tedious history of the 1960s and 1970s fashion, but Trina knows it's all really about loving the clothes. LOVE, man, that's still the answer.

Richard Martin
Curator, The Costume Institute
The Metropolitan Museum of Art

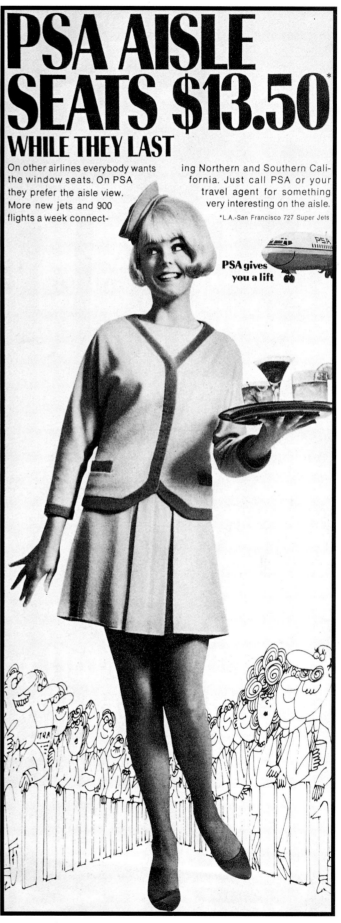

A groovy PSA airline stewardess from *Look* magazine, November 26, 1968.

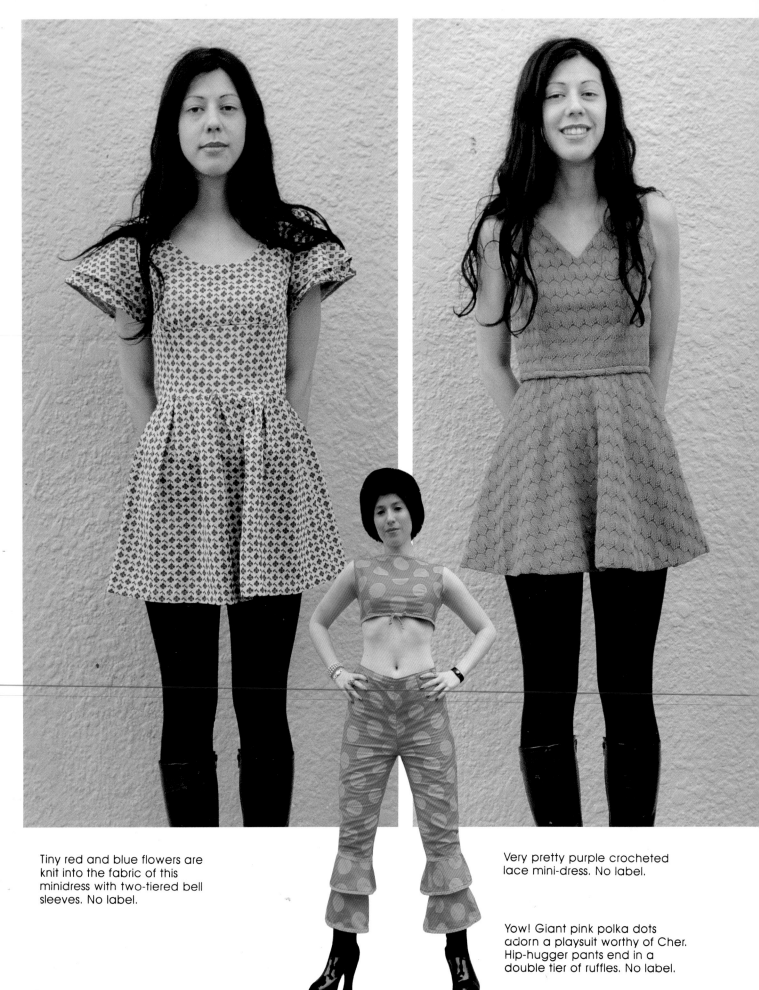

Tiny red and blue flowers are knit into the fabric of this minidress with two-tiered bell sleeves. No label.

Very pretty purple crocheted lace mini-dress. No label.

Yow! Giant pink polka dots adorn a playsuit worthy of Cher. Hip-hugger pants end in a double tier of ruffles. No label.

Introduction

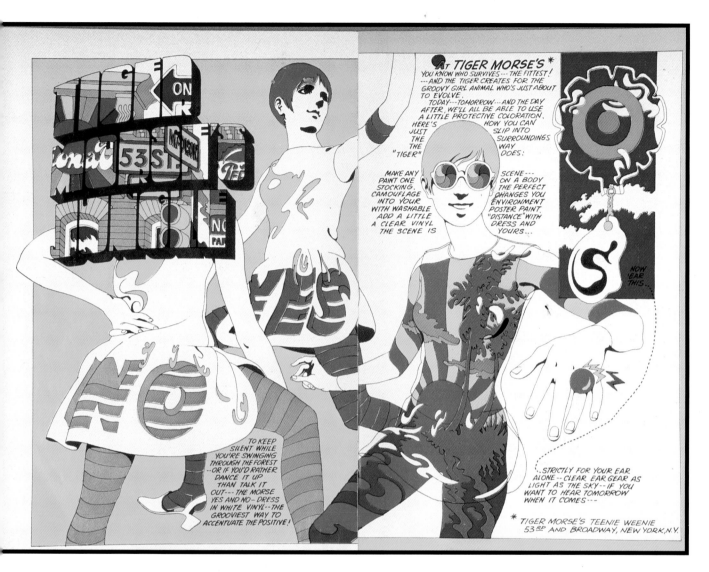

An advertisement for Tiger Morse's New York boutique from the comic book *Mod Love*, 1967.

There's a saying about fashion that a five year old dress is considered dowdy, a ten year old dress is hideous, a twenty year old dress is hilarious, but when the dress turns thirty, it's beautiful all over again. That's one reason fashions from the 1960s and 1970s are so very hot today, when once you couldn't give them away.

Another reason for the sudden popularity of clothes from this period is that - let's face it - there's almost nothing left in decent condition from earlier periods - the 1950s and earlier - and what is left is selling at sky-high prices in vintage clothing stores. If you have the good luck to find that lovely little tailored rayon dress from the '40s at a flea market, at an affordable price, chances are it's hopelessly stained under the arms (anti-

perspirants hadn't been perfected yet) or some idiot took the hem up in the '60s, and cut off the excess material so it can't be restored. If the dress was made of silk, your chances of finding it in wearable condition are even worse. Instead of mere staining under the arms, the fabric's probably rotted away! As a result, vintage clothing stores that scorned clothing from the '60s and '70s as short a time ago as 1990, now feature wall-to-wall polyester.

Here's another reason; today's young taste-makers grew up in the '70s and they remember that period with fond nostalgia. That's the reason for the success of such movies as *The Brady Bunch*; generation Xers watched and loved the TV show as children. Now they're out in the big scary world, trying to be responsible grownups. Why shouldn't they return, at least in fun, to a time when they felt safe and loved, and their only responsibility was to put away their Barbie® and Skipper® dolls, and get their homework done in time to watch "Charlie's Angels?"

Those of us over thirty share the same warm nostalgia for the sixties, that psychedelic era of Beatles, Hippies and be-ins, and the fabulous clothes we danced in.

Finally, fashions from the '60s and '70s are still comparatively available; although growing harder to find and more expensive every day, they can still be found for a few dollars at flea markets, thrift shops and garage sales. They're also very wearable today, when the hottest new fashions are mere copies of outfits from thirty years before, yet cost over twice as much as you would pay for the original garment at a vintage clothing store.

Labels are often long-gone from older garments, but if they remain and are readable, here are some names to look for (More about some of these designers later in this book!): anything British, especially if it's from Carnaby Street or Biba's; clothes from famous 1960s stores or boutiques like Tiger Morse's; Young Edwardian and Young Innocents, both by Arpeja; Lilly Pulitzer; Diane Von Furstenberg; any famous designers such as Oscar De La Renta or Rudy Gernreich; anything at all by Pucci, even underwear; and Betsey, Bunkie and Nini or Alley Cat, which were Betsey Johnson's earlier labels. I once heard a woman at a vintage clothing shop say that Betsey Johnson was the Mercedes of used clothing; her fashions are always in demand.

When you start collecting clothes from the '60s and '70s, you'll notice certain differences between them and contemporary clothes, or between them and earlier clothes. One is the zippers. Dresses from the '40s and early '50s all have side zippers. By the end of the '50s, long back zippers were introduced so that women with high, teased beehive hairdos could step into the dresses, rather than having to pull them on over their heads and waste all that hair spray. By the '60s, long back zippers were here to stay, and all dresses from that period have them.

Another difference is the hems. To put it simply, 25 year-old-dresses are better made than today's dresses; they have big hems, today's dresses have none. What passes for a hem these days is a tiny machine-sewn roll at the bottom of the dress.

You'll also notice that your vintage dresses are made in America and boast a union label, whereas too many of today's fashions are manufactured somewhere in Outer Slobbovia by children who are paid 20 cents a day, and the clothes show it. Their buttons fall off after one wearing and the seams rip. The conclusion? Not only are the older dresses better made (remember those hems?), but the '60s and '70s were a more prosperous time for Americans. It doesn't take a rocket scientist to make the connection between better clothes, better times, and the union label.

How to wear vintage outfits from the '60s and '70s? Well, slim young women in their 20s can get away with almost anything. Shopping at my local supermarket, I saw a young woman who was wearing an entire '60s outfit: mini dress, vintage tote bag, lace tights and white vinyl go-go boots, and she looked great. If you're 40 or over, though, watch out — you don't want to look like a bag lady who is still wearing her original 30 year old wardrobe! I recommend one fabulous vintage item mixed with contemporary accessories. In the end, however, your final decision, when buying a garment from the '60s and '70s, or from any other period, should be based on how much you love it. Then, wear and enjoy!

Chapter One

The Care & Feeding of Polyester

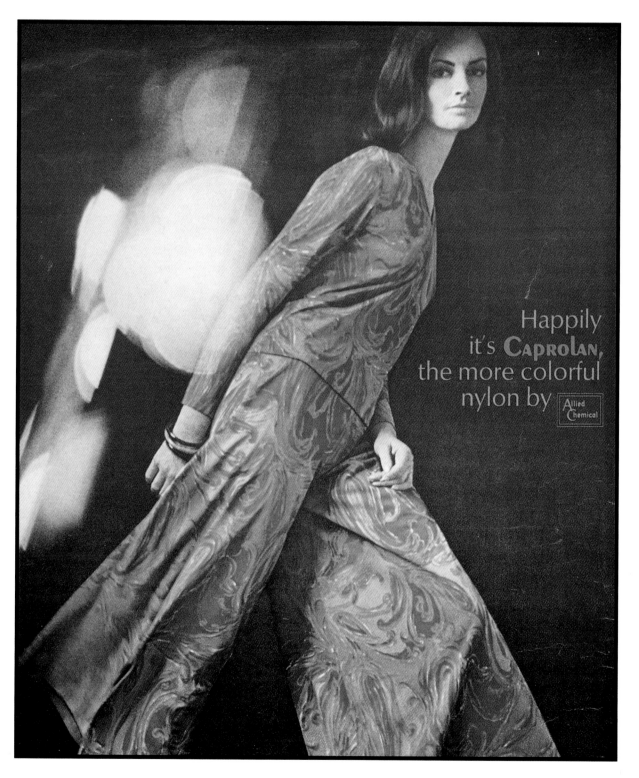

Advertisement for Caprolan nylon from *Vogue*, April 15,

Synthetic fabrics have actually been around much longer than you think. As early as 1884, French inventor Hilaire De Chardonnet created a silk substitute, made from wood pulp. "Chardonnet silk", as it was then called, had a great many faults - among other things, it was highly flammable. The unfortunate *fin de siecle* women must have gone up like torches. By 1924, the garment industry was using an improved form of Chardonnet's invention, and calling it "rayon." The new rayon was still not perfect - it tended to shrink, and was not colorfast (this is still a problem with much of today's rayon clothing), but it was a good, cheap substitute for silk.

Then, in 1931, Wallace Hume Carothers, working for the duPont Company, produced nylon, the first successful synthetic fiber made from oil refinery by-products, or petrochemicals. By 1938, nylon stockings manufactured by duPont were on the market. Unfortunately for women, nylon was diverted to military use during World War II. Stronger than silk, it replaced that fabric in parachutes, and was woven into heavy "flak jackets" that protected against shell fragments. During World War II, when the more desirable silk and nylon were unavailable, nylon was used widely also in civilian clothing for men and women.

Women got their nylon back after the war, and the long lines and mob scenes at postwar nylon stocking sales attested to its desirability. Soon new petrochemical fabrics followed, and the late forties and fifties saw the growing popularity of garments fashioned from synthetic fabrics with brand names like Dacron®, Orlon®, Fortrel®, and Kodel®. The term "drip-dry" entered the English language; people loved the new fabrics that you didn't have to iron and sweaters that were machine washable. (Some sweaters from that period bore labels that boasted "100% Virgin Orlon"!)

The general public tends to lump all synthetic fabrics together under the name polyester, but in fact there are many different synthetics. Acetate, for instance, was actually the second man-made fiber produced in America, and was originally considered a type of rayon. Acrylic was developed by the duPont Company in 1944. Orlon is an acrylic fabric, while Dacron, Fortrel, and Kodel are polyesters. In this book, just to simplify things, when the content label on a garment is missing but I know that the fabric is man-made, I've decided to call it polyester.

Dacron® polyester was introduced in 1953 and Kodel® polyester in 1958. Polyester really came into its own in the 1960s, and is forever

Fiber	These Blend Levels Give Excellent Performance	Comments
Polyester: Dacron Fortrel Kodel Vycron	50 to 65% with cotton or linen 55% with rayon	Excellent wrinkle-resistance—the best of all man-made fibers
Acrylic: Acrilan Creslan Orlon Zefran	80% with cotton 70% with rayon	Very good wrinkle-resistance
Nylon	100%	Tricots and knits are best
Arnel	100%	Noted for good pleatability

Chart from April, 1964, *Good Housekeeping*, explaining the different types of synthetic fabrics.

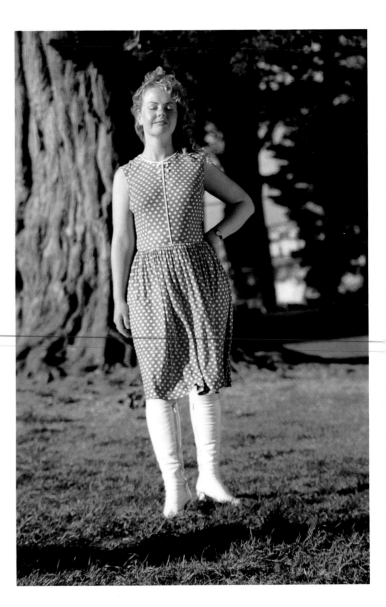

100% Arnel triacetate dress from the early 1960s.

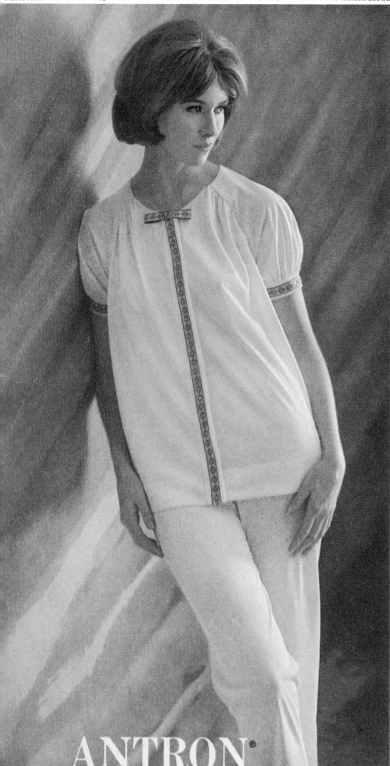

Advertisement for Antron nylon, from *Good Housekeeping*, April, 1964.

associated with that decade. It was a perfect choice for the futuristic image of the 1960s. Literally made of a plastic, it was a miracle fabric. It reproduced the bright, sometimes day-glow colors of that decade beautifully, and never ran or faded. It didn't fray, either, and the hems of many garments from the '60s and '70s were left raw for that reason. Dacron could be knit or woven, and the shiny threads were so slippery that most stains simply washed out. It could even be made to imitate wool or cotton (or even fur!), or be combined with those natural fabrics. Unlike rayon, it didn't wrinkle, and you didn't have to iron it.

In fact, whatever you do, never iron polyester or any other petrochemical synthetic with a hot iron unless you want to see cloth melt and turn into hard plastic! If the polyester mini-dress you just dug out of a pile at the flea market is dreadfully wrinkled, throw it into the washer, using cold water. It will emerge in perfect shape. If absolutely necessary, you may touch it up with a warm, not hot, iron.

Polyester, like the plastic it comes from, doesn't decay, so, unlike silks or rayons, you won't find beautiful thirty year old dresses with the cloth rotted away. And, of course, moths don't eat it. The human race may eventually become extinct, but cockroaches and polyester will remain on this planet forever.

You may come across a wonderful polyester garment with cuts or tears in the fabric; it happens to everything. If those bellbottoms with a rip in the knee are otherwise too good a find to pass up, look for ways to patch them. Does the garment have a big hem (most clothing from that period had big hems). Is it so long that you'll need to take it up anyway? Does it have pockets, especially deep ones? Material taken from pockets or the hem will make good patches; in the case of prints, try to match the design of the print. And save any leftover fabric for possible future patches!

As for stains, as mentioned above, many stains easily come out of polyester. I usually squeeze a good dollop of dishwashing liquid onto the stain and rub it in, then let the garment sit for about an hour before putting it into the washing machine.

Ironically, rayon has become a very desirable fabric today, despite the fact that it requires costly dry-cleaning, while wondrously washable polyester went out of favor in the earthtone eighties. A friend who simply refuses to wear polyester tells me, "It doesn't breathe." That's okay with me. As long as I can breathe, it doesn't matter to me whether or not my dress can! Of course I don't recommend polyester for every-thing, everyday. Wool will keep you warmer, cotton is crisper and more traditional, silks and rayons are - well, silkier. But you wouldn't want to wear any of them all the time; for instance, you wouldn't wear wool in hot weather. Bright, unpretentious polyester has its place; for one thing, it's downright fun.

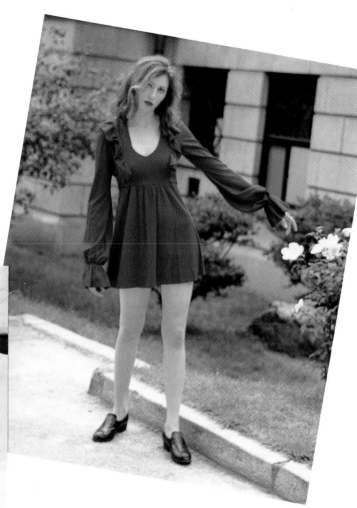

Poetic mini-dress made from maroon synthetic jersey. Label reads, "Bishop's Sportswear."

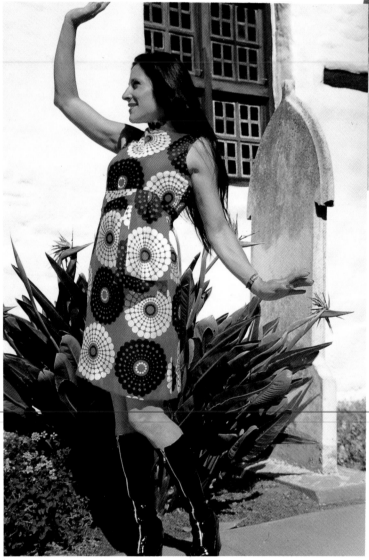

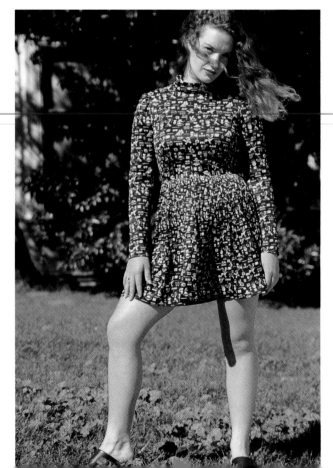

Red, white, and blue mini-dress made from unknown synthetic fiber. Label reads, "Morton Miles for Jeunesse, New York."

Very short mini-dress made from 100% Arnel triacetate, permanently pleated at the hip. The fabric design is a Dutch motif on dark blue. "E.D. Juniors of San Francisco."

Dacron.
Red, white & new!

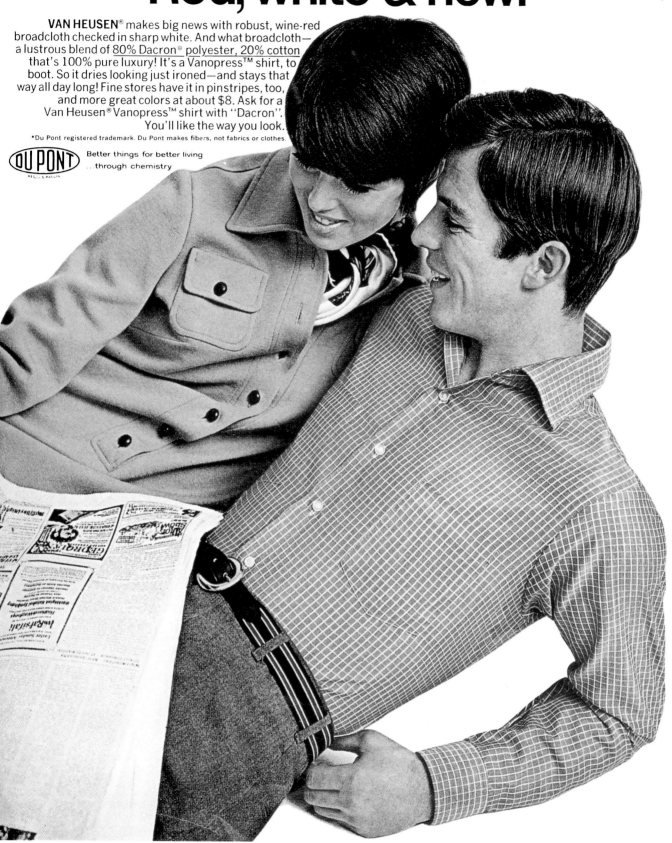

VAN HEUSEN® makes big news with robust, wine-red broadcloth checked in sharp white. And what broadcloth— a lustrous blend of <u>80% Dacron* polyester, 20% cotton</u> that's 100% pure luxury! It's a Vanopress™ shirt, to boot. So it dries looking just ironed—and stays that way all day long! Fine stores have it in pinstripes, too, and more great colors at about $8. Ask for a Van Heusen® Vanopress™ shirt with "Dacron". You'll like the way you look.

*Du Pont registered trademark. Du Pont makes fibers, not fabrics or clothes.

DU PONT
REG. U.S. PAT. OFF.

Better things for better living
...through chemistry

Advertisement for Dacron, from *Look*, November 26, 1968.

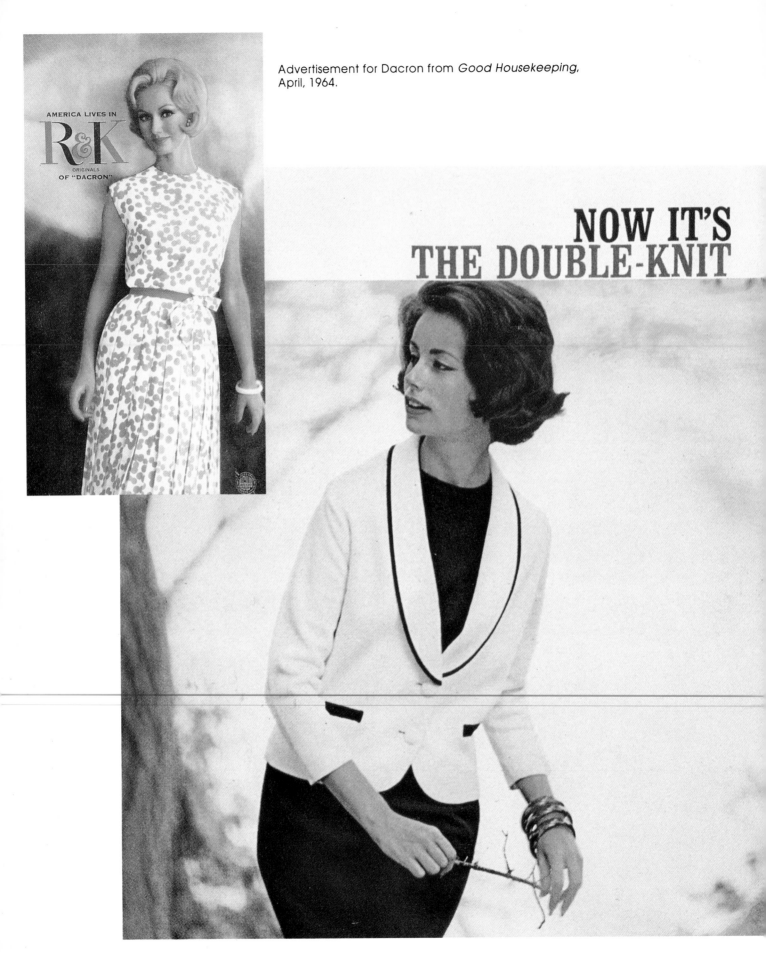

Advertisement for Dacron from *Good Housekeeping*,
April, 1964.

AMERICA LIVES IN
R&K
ORIGINALS
OF "DACRON"

NOW IT'S
THE DOUBLE-KNIT

Advertisement for Orlon double-knit, from *Glamour*,
November, 1961.

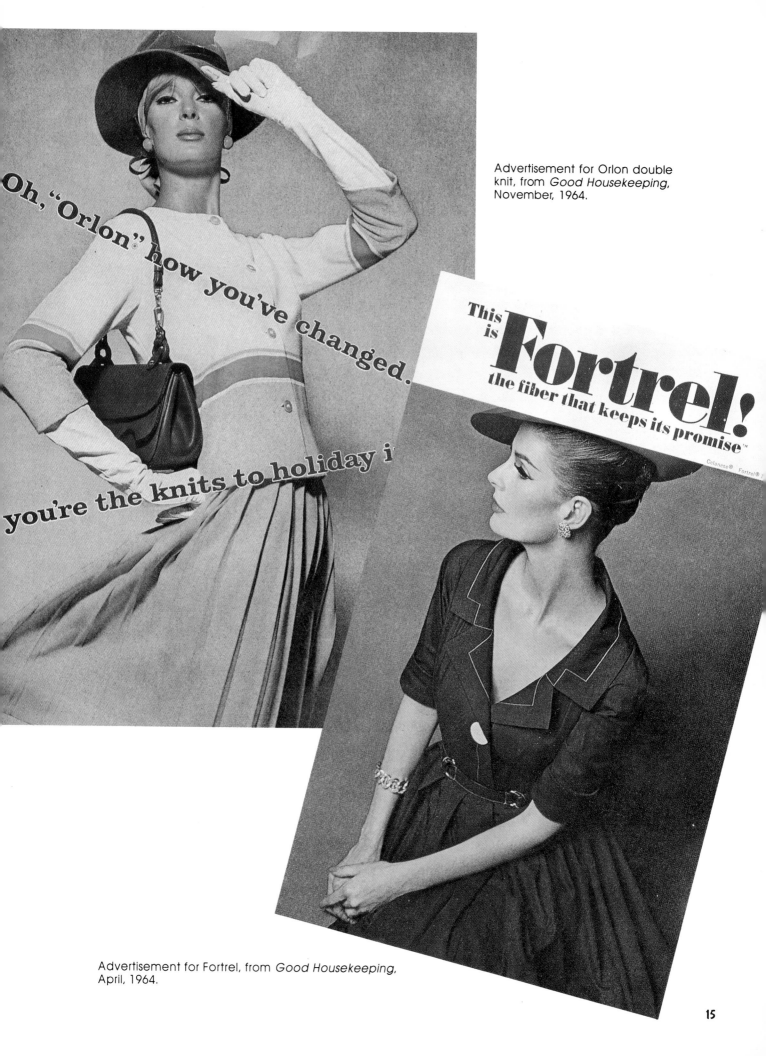

Oh, "Orlon" how you've changed.

you're the knits to holiday i

Advertisement for Orlon double knit, from *Good Housekeeping*, November, 1964.

This is **Fortrel!** the fiber that keeps its promise™

Celanese® Fortrel®

Advertisement for Fortrel, from *Good Housekeeping*, April, 1964.

15

Chapter Two

Jackie Oh!

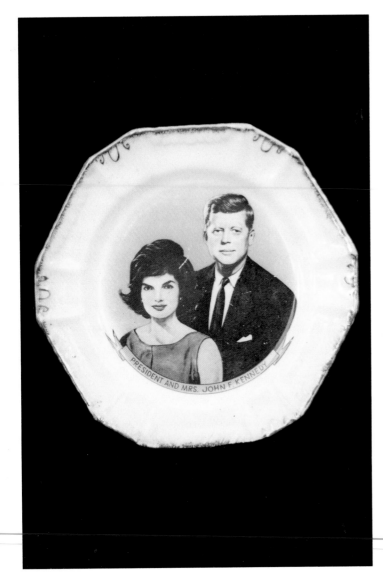

Jack and Jackie on a plate. Royal Tara fine bone china, made in Ireland.

At the beginning of the 1960s, the ultimate icon for women was Jacqueline Kennedy, the most beautiful and fashionable First Lady this country has ever had (at least since Dolly Madison). Her ladylike appearance inspired thousands of women to adopt her flip hairstyle and chic A-line dresses. From the start of that decade, and for the next thirty years, no magazine was considered complete without its requisite article on "Jackie." The cover article for the April, 1964 issue of *Good Housekeeping* magazine was "Jacqueline Kennedy: The Future of a Noble Lady." Their November, 1964 issue featured not one, but two articles on Jackie: "How I Hope He'll Be Remembered," by Jacqueline Kennedy herself, and "Jackie Kennedy and Her Children: One Year After the Tragedy." Meanwhile, the June 30, 1964 issue of *Look* magazine featured "The Kennedy Legend." *Teen Time* got into the act with such articles as "Jackie Kennedy's Teenage Loves," in their December, 1962, issue.

The clothes that Jackie wore in the early '60s were not very different from what women had been wearing in the '50s: "nice girl" dresses with peter pan collars and bouffant skirts. Only their new, shorter length distinguished them from the fashions of the previous decade. The January, 1961 issue of *Seventeen* magazine heralded the new skirt length in an article called "short-stop Skirt: American as apple pie (and just as popular): the new, brief, just-above-the-knee skirt — a sporting look that's here to stay." Rather than "here to stay," of course, this was just the beginning. When Jackie shortened her skirts in 1965, so did millions of other American women, and the mini skirt arrived, but not without controversy. Some countries passed laws against the mini, and mini skirts were banned in the Vatican. Nonetheless, hemlines were to creep higher and higher throughout the sixties, almost up to there, before they fell all the way back down at the end of the decade.

At the beginning of the decade, waistlines, too, were where they had been for the past thirty years — right at the waist; but that started changing pretty quickly. The April, 1964 *Good Housekeeping* shows an A-line dress that skims the waist, like the kind we now associate with Jackie Kennedy, and features a knee-length shift with no waist at all. Within a few years, waistlines would drop to the hips in a style reminiscent of the roaring '20s, rise up to below the bust in a sometimes-'30s-retro style, sometimes true Empire (gathered directly beneath the bust) for the first time in about 150 years. Or the waist would disappear entirely — it would be anywhere but at the true waistline!

The fashionable lady at the beginning of the 1960s, complete with hat, gloves, purse and nylons, from an advertisement in *Glamour*, November, 1961.

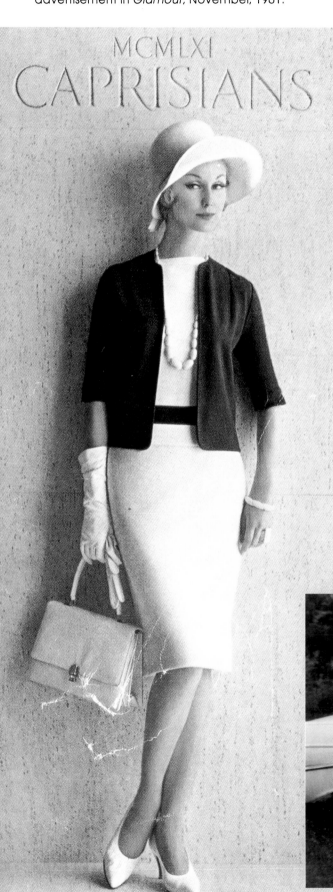

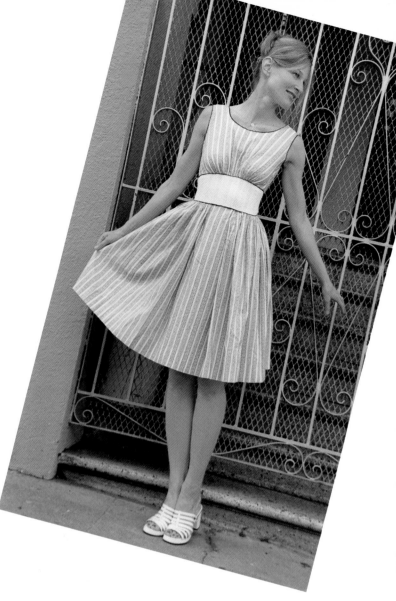

Black and white cotton sundress with black rick-rack trim.

Danette's mom and dad in 1961. She is wearing the cotton sundress with the rick-rack trim.

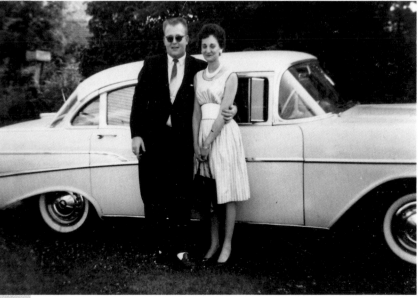

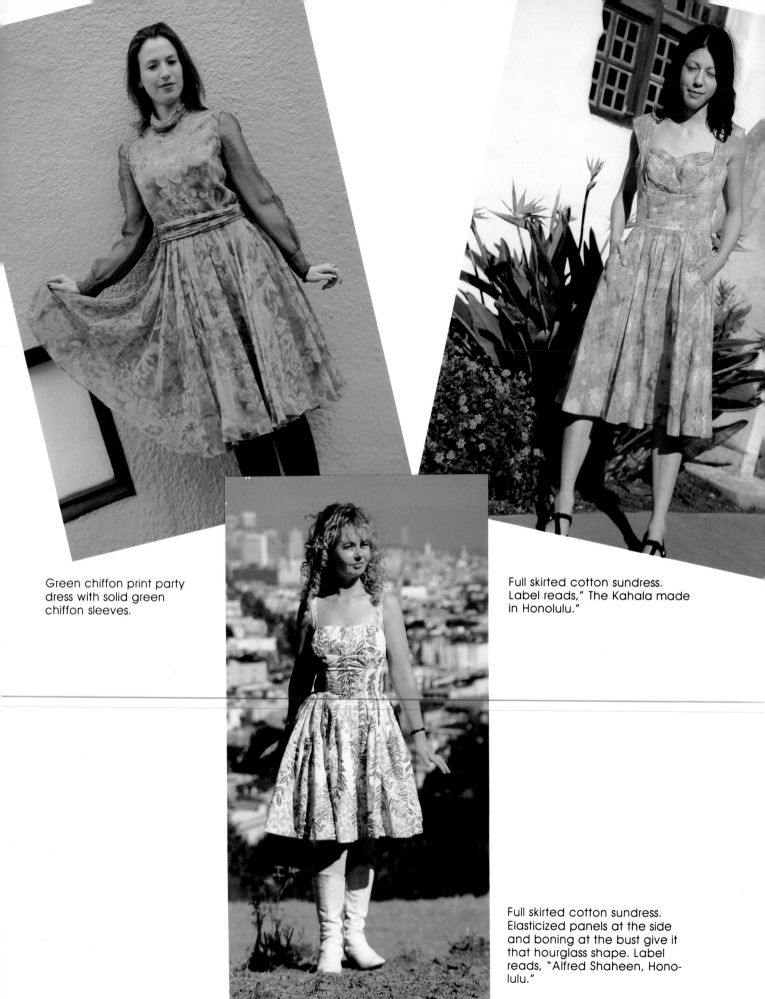

Green chiffon print party dress with solid green chiffon sleeves.

Full skirted cotton sundress. Label reads," The Kahala made in Honolulu."

Full skirted cotton sundress. Elasticized panels at the side and boning at the bust give it that hourglass shape. Label reads, "Alfred Shaheen, Honolulu."

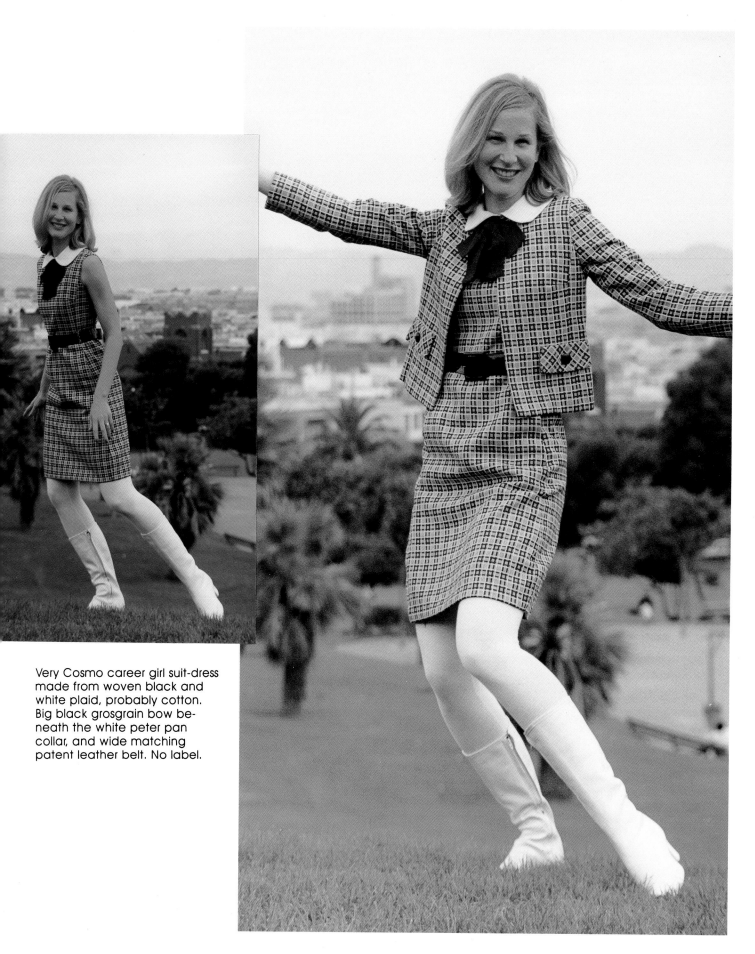

Very Cosmo career girl suit-dress made from woven black and white plaid, probably cotton. Big black grosgrain bow beneath the white peter pan collar, and wide matching patent leather belt. No label.

The same dress with its matching jacket. The faux pocket flaps are trimmed with big black buttons.

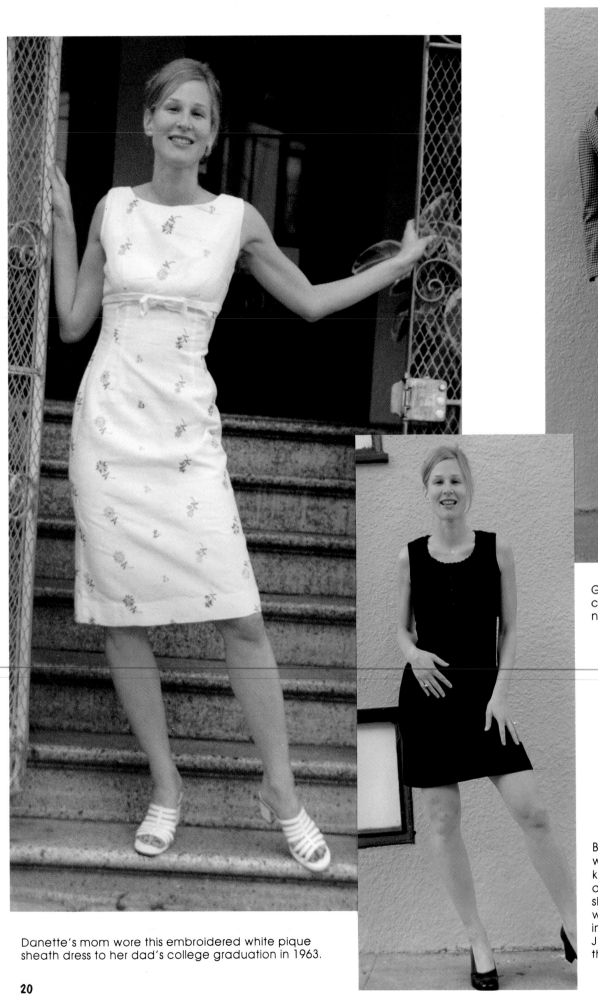

Green wool
checked suit,
no label.

Black 100%
wool double-
knit sheath
dress, worn
shorter than it
was originally
intended. "For
J.P.s only", says
the label.

Danette's mom wore this embroidered white pique
sheath dress to her dad's college graduation in 1963.

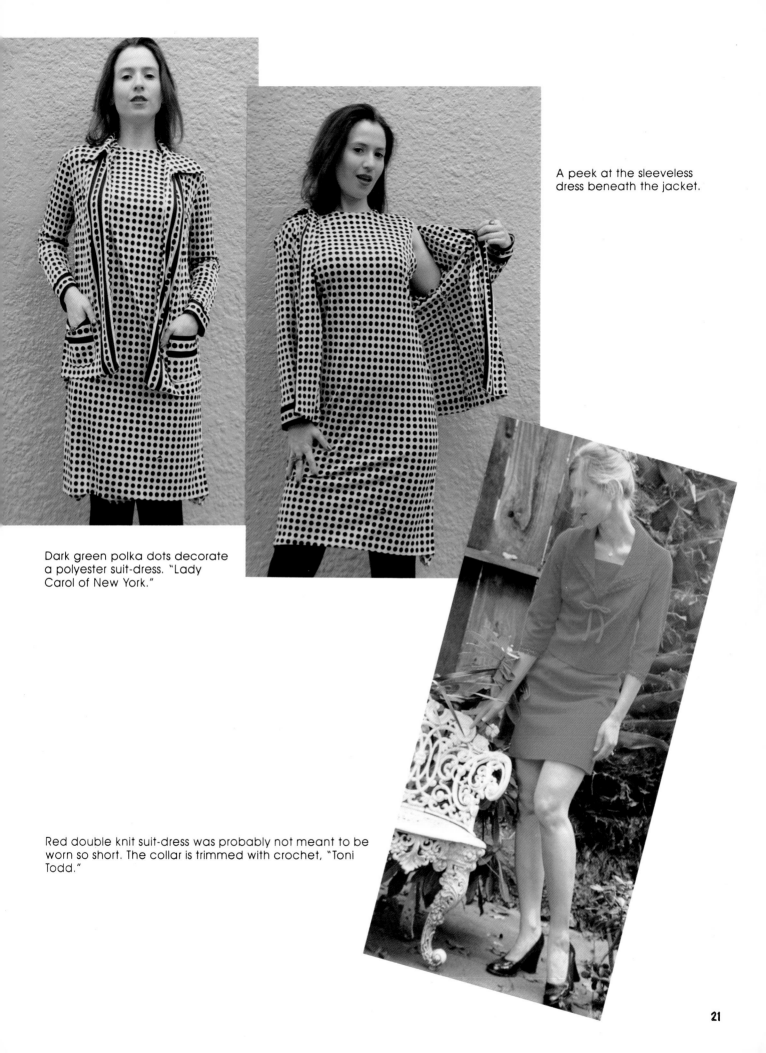

A peek at the sleeveless dress beneath the jacket.

Dark green polka dots decorate a polyester suit-dress. "Lady Carol of New York."

Red double knit suit-dress was probably not meant to be worn so short. The collar is trimmed with crochet, "Toni Todd."

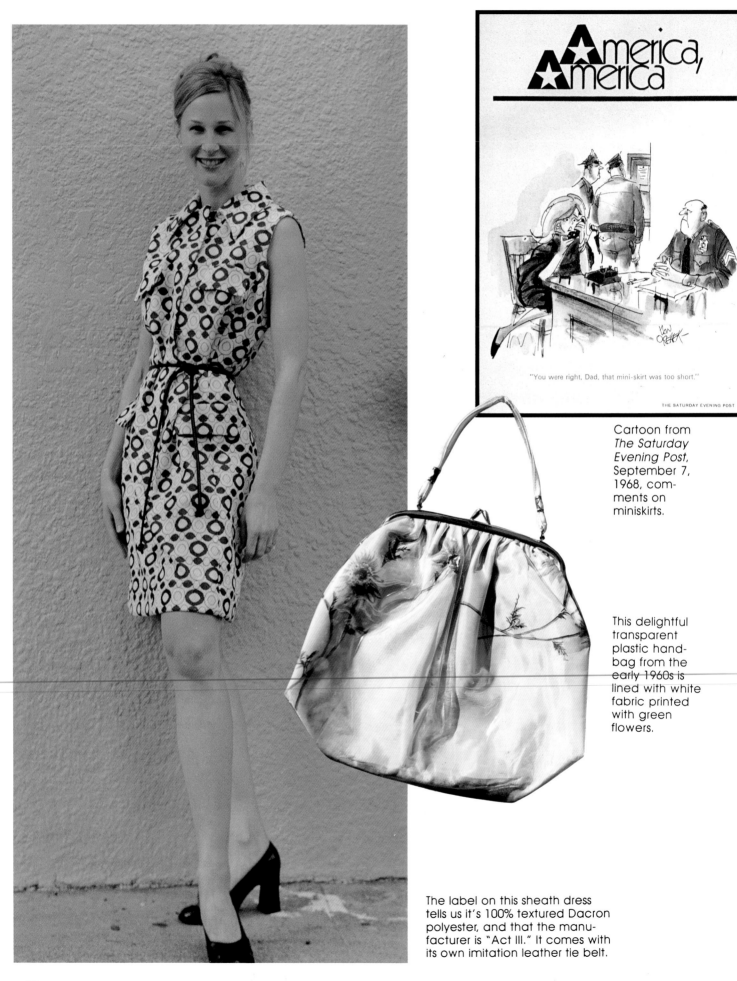

"You were right, Dad, that mini-skirt was too short."

THE SATURDAY EVENING POST

Cartoon from
The Saturday Evening Post,
September 7,
1968, comments on
miniskirts.

This delightful transparent plastic handbag from the early 1960s is lined with white fabric printed with green flowers.

The label on this sheath dress tells us it's 100% textured Dacron polyester, and that the manufacturer is "Act III." It comes with its own imitation leather tie belt.

22

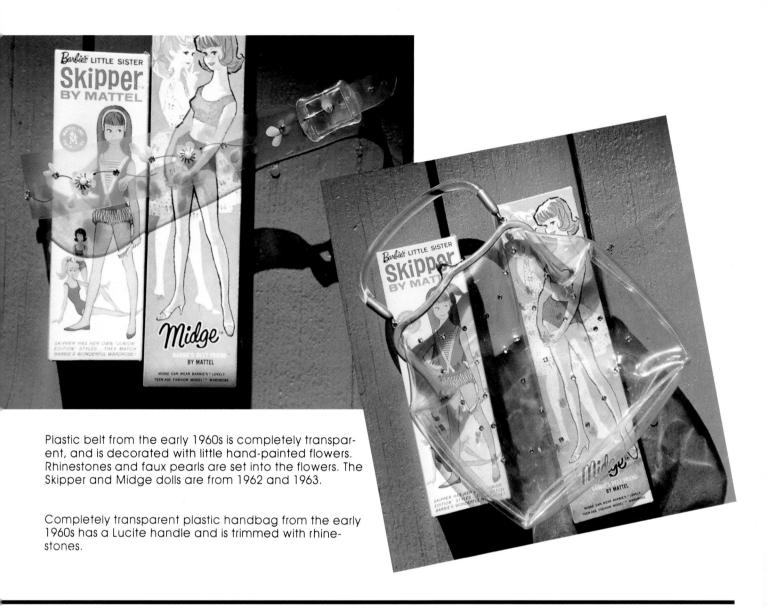

Plastic belt from the early 1960s is completely transparent, and is decorated with little hand-painted flowers. Rhinestones and faux pearls are set into the flowers. The Skipper and Midge dolls are from 1962 and 1963.

Completely transparent plastic handbag from the early 1960s has a Lucite handle and is trimmed with rhinestones.

Gingham

Brigitte Bardot, the sex symbol of the late '50s and early '60s, wore a pink gingham dress for her second wedding in 1959. By 1960, knockoffs of that dress, and other gingham styles, were being worn by millions of American women. Gingham carried with it an old-fashioned, country girl air of innocence. In a world whose citizens lived in the shadow of The Bomb, perhaps the sweetness and simplicity suggested by gingham provided a much-needed escape. Whatever the reason, the passion for gingham presaged the return to organic simplicity that would soon take the country by storm.

Gingham dress by "Vicky Vaughn" from an advertisement in *Seventeen*, January, 1961.

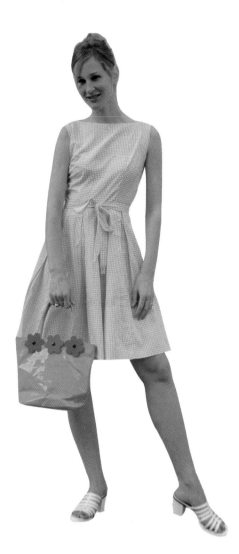

Orange gingham sundress. The orange handbag is contemporary, from 1996.

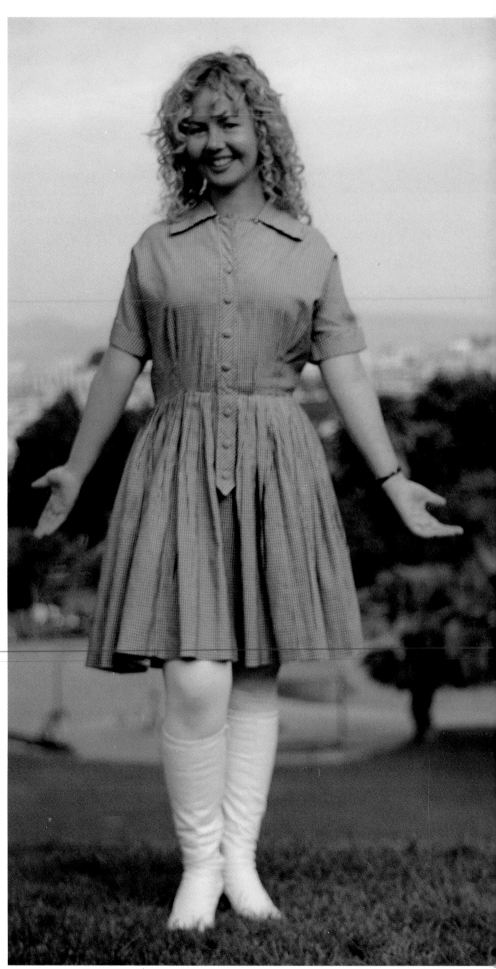

Black and white gingham shirt-dress. The row of buttons down the front are faux; it zips up the back with a metal zipper. Later, most zippers were plastic. "A Pomette Fashion."

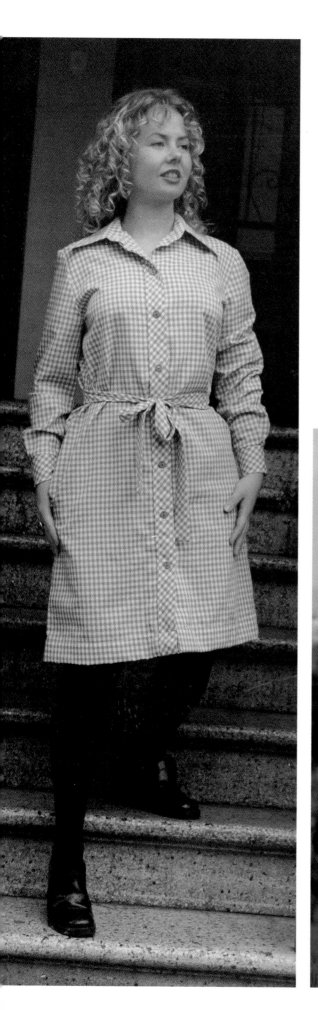

Green gingham shirt-dress with self tie-belt. "Designed and tailored by Gordon of Philadelphia."

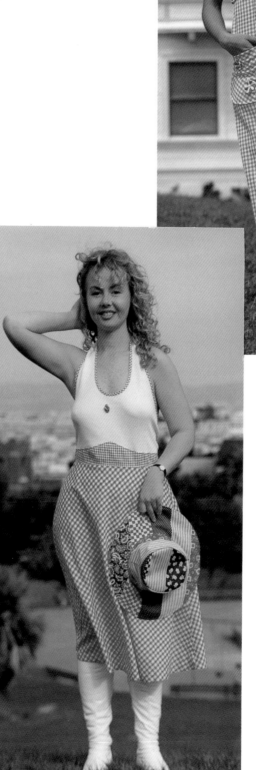

This dress, with white pique top and long red gingham skirt, is a favorite. Crocheted red daisies trim the top, the big patch pockets, and circle the high waist. "Alice of California, permapress."

Sundress with a big red gingham skirt has small gingham checks at the waist and binding the white knit top, upon which is appliquéd a tiny bouquet of flowers. The label says, "Jody T of California", and tells us it's made of 65% polyester and 35% cotton.

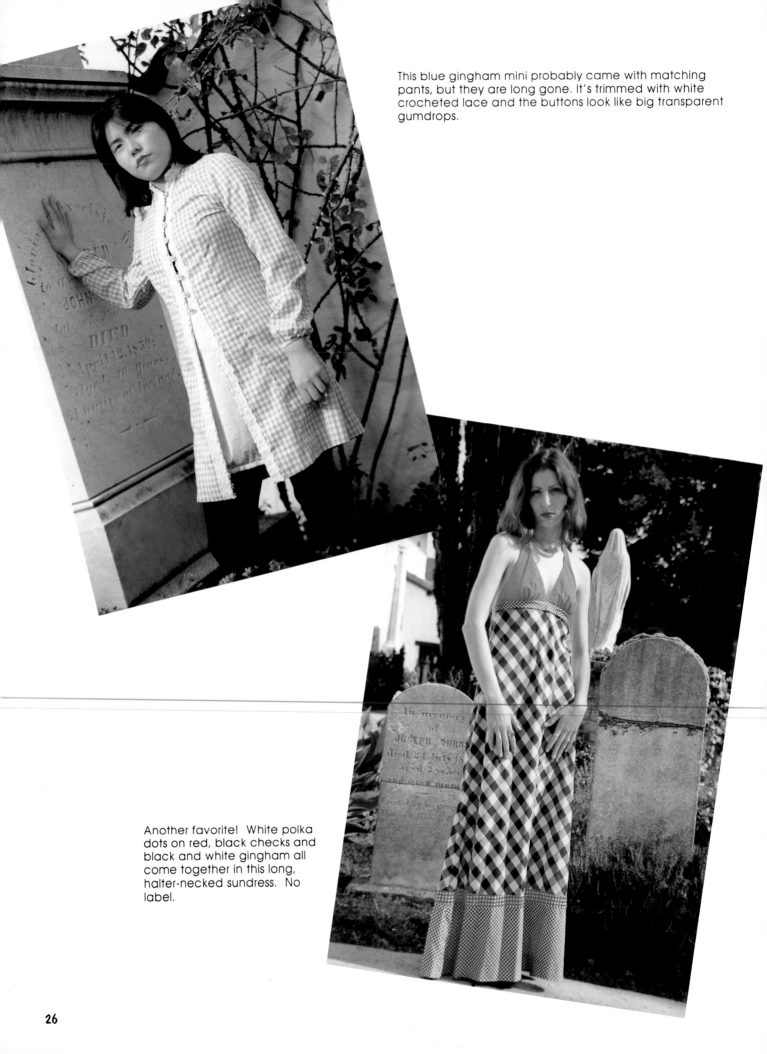

This blue gingham mini probably came with matching pants, but they are long gone. It's trimmed with white crocheted lace and the buttons look like big transparent gumdrops.

Another favorite! White polka dots on red, black checks and black and white gingham all come together in this long, halter-necked sundress. No label.

The Shirtdress

Shirtdresses are simple, tailored dresses cut like a man's shirt and buttoned down the front. At the beginning of the '60s, shirtdressess, despite their tailoring, featured knee-high full skirts and cinched waists. Often the collar was a Peter Pan style and the sleeves were made to be rolled up to three-quarters length. By the end of the decade, the collar had grown long and pointy and instead of a tight waist and full skirt the shirtdress had become a mini shift, worn straight up and down or with its own self belt or chain belt. Sometimes the shirtdress was interpreted as a flattering long dress. By the early '70s, although the waistline had returned, the shirtdress was no longer cinched tightly; the dress now skimmed the figure and the A-line skirt ended just below the knee. Through each period, with changes in skirt length and styling, the shirtdress remained classic and wearable, now as then.

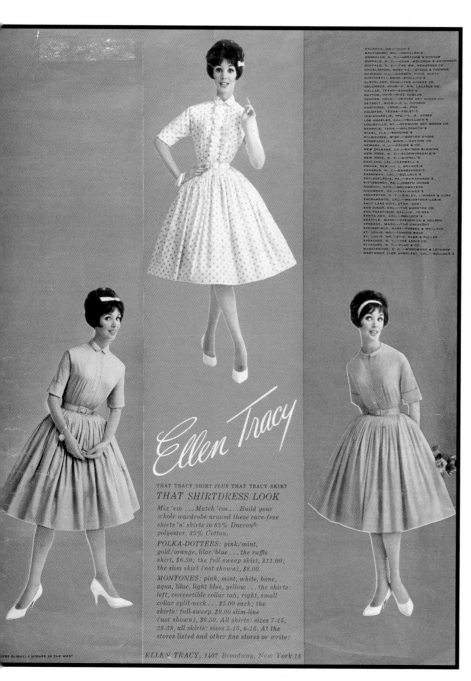

Advertisement for Ellen Tracy shirt-dresses from *Seventeen*, January, 1961.

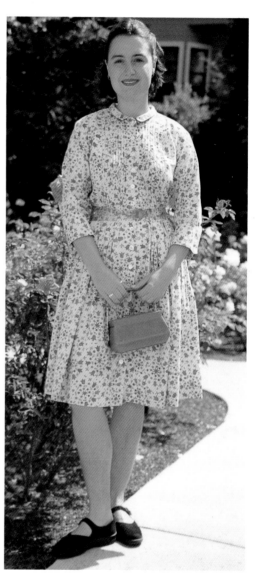

A proper little cotton shirt-dress from the early 1960s, printed with Pennsylvania Dutch designs. The label says, "Sue Brett junior dress."

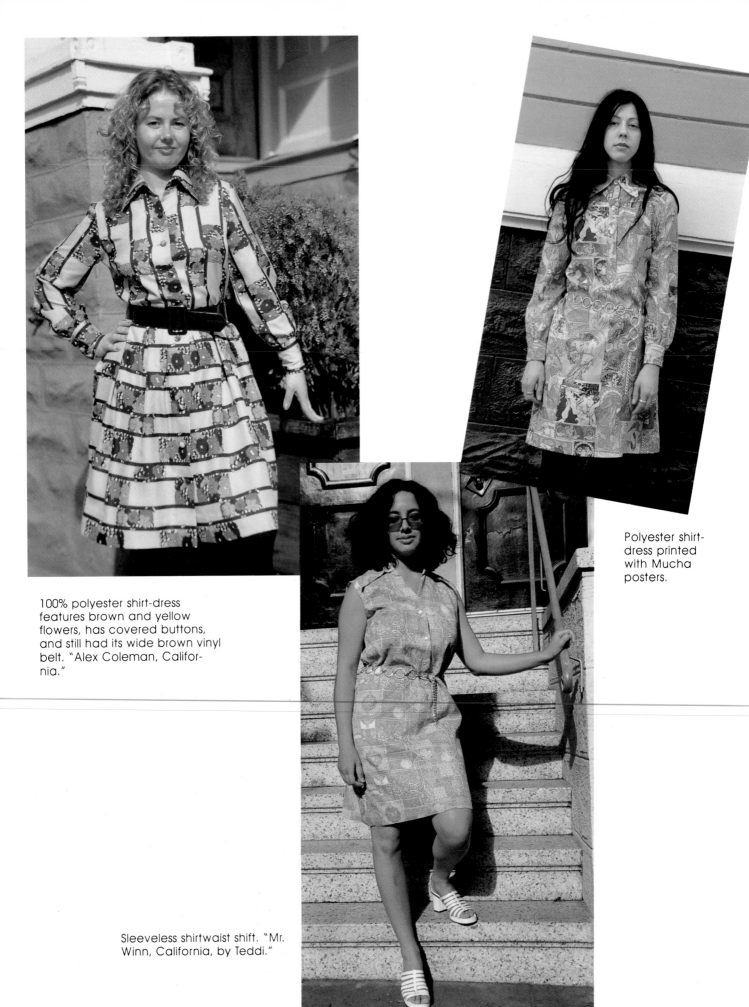

Polyester shirt-dress printed with Mucha posters.

100% polyester shirt-dress features brown and yellow flowers, has covered buttons, and still had its wide brown vinyl belt. "Alex Coleman, California."

Sleeveless shirtwaist shift. "Mr. Winn, California, by Teddi."

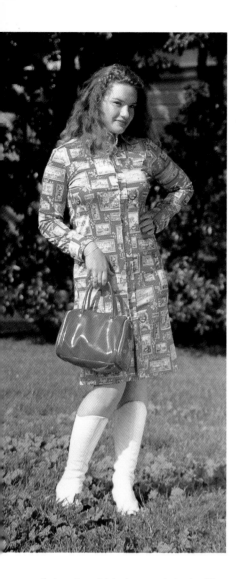

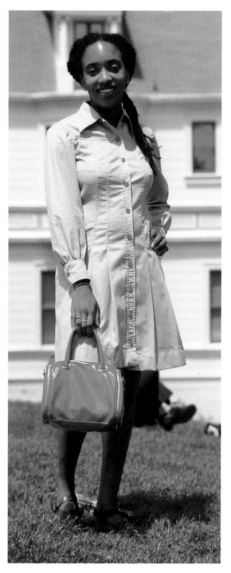

Shirt-dress has pleats top-stitched in red to match the red buttons and red with white pin dots lining the collar and cuffs. The fabric is narrow blue and white stripes, and the label says, "Lord and Taylor."

Polyester shirt-dress printed with French Art Nouveau wine labels. Label says, "Shirtmaker."

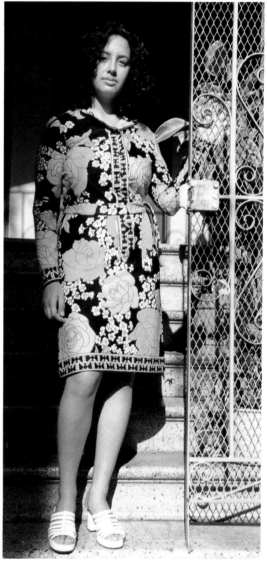

Giant yellow and beige roses on a black background cover this shirtwaist-styled shift with its own self-tie belt. The label says it's from Joseph Magnin's, a big San Francisco department store that no longer exists.

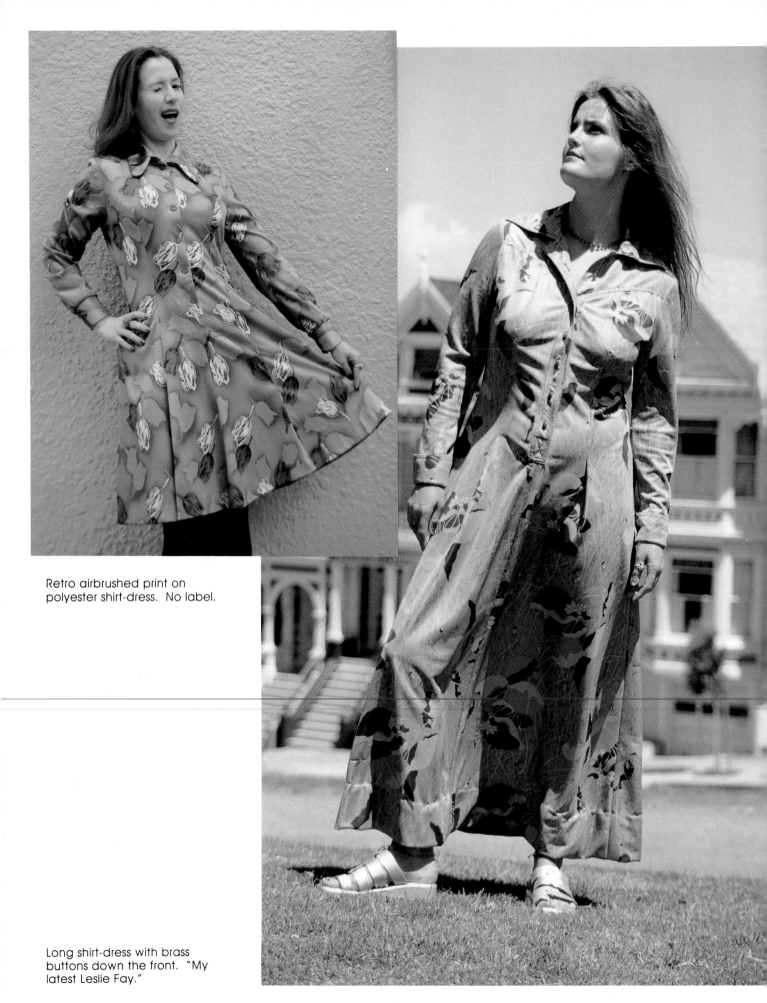

Retro airbrushed print on
polyester shirt-dress. No label.

Long shirt-dress with brass
buttons down the front. "My
latest Leslie Fay."

30

The Ubiquitous Daisy

As symbols of the anti-war movement and "flower children" who demonstrated for peace, daisies sprang up like, well, daisies, throughout the '60s. The perky little flowers could be seen on art, advertising, and clothes. They became associated with perky young actresses like Marlo Thomas and Mary Tyler Moore, and some who were not so young, but were still perky, like Doris Day.

Long 100% polyester shirt-dress printed in bright pinks and oranges. "Kiyomi Hawaii, Liberty House."

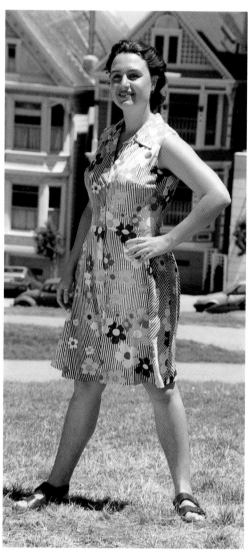

Orange, gold, blue, and white daisies scattered over dark green stripes. Gold metal buttons down the front. No label.

Very bright purple, pink, and green print looks great under black light. This long shirt-dress has a self-tie belt, and the label reads "Beeline Fashions." Printing on the selvage of the material tells us that it's "THC Hawaiian textiles #9318."

Yellow patch pockets match the daisies marching up and down the stripes on this high-waisted cotton sundress. It zips up the front and the label says "Gilead."

Long rows of daisies in bright orange, pink and yellow decorate this cotton jumpsuit with very wide legs and patch pockets. No label.

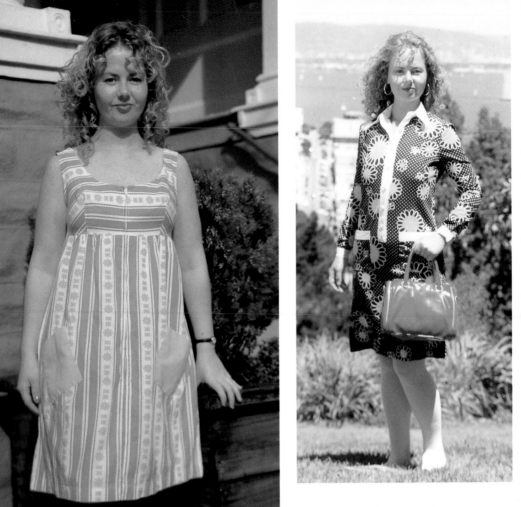

Cotton shirt-dress with white collar, cuffs and front button panel, decorated with daisies and white polka dots. The label reads "Craely" and tells us it came from I. Magnin & Co., a former San Francisco department store.

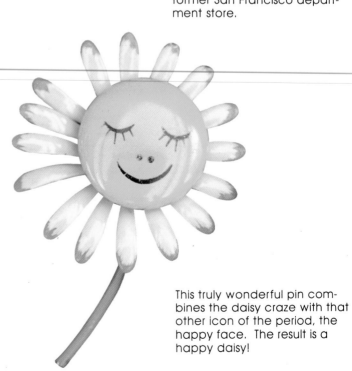

This truly wonderful pin combines the daisy craze with that other icon of the period, the happy face. The result is a happy daisy!

Chapter Three
The Shift

Once waistlines were done away with, the basic shape of the sixties became the shift, a dress reminiscent of the flapper fashions of the 1920s. Originally knee length and hanging straight down from the shoulders to the knees, the hem shortened as the '60s progressed until it became a micro-mini. Sometimes the shift was made from stretch fabrics, in which case, instead of hanging straight down from the shoulders, it moulded itself to the figure. These styles look great if you are 15 and have the right figure. Since its lines were so simple, the shift was perfectly suited to bright, almost day-glow psychedelic prints and Pucci-inspired abstracts or the ubiquitous daisies and polka dots of the '60s.

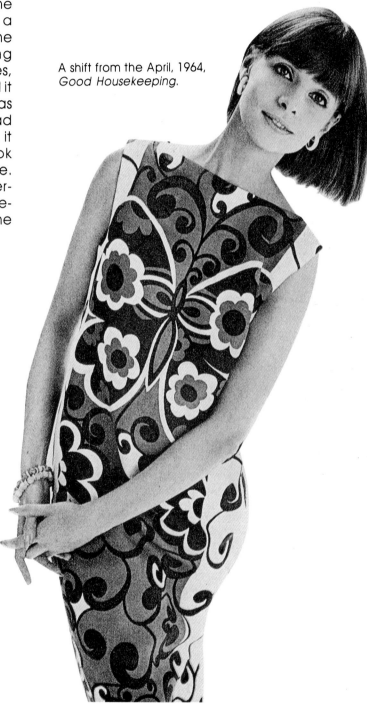

A shift from the April, 1964, *Good Housekeeping.*

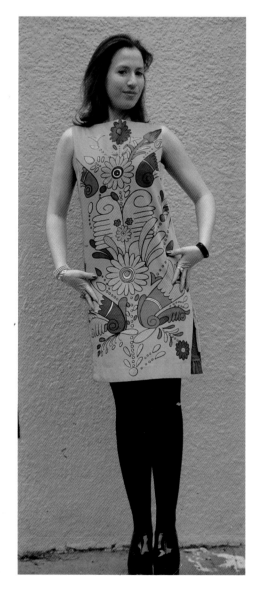

A cotton, bateau-necked shift very like the one pictured in *Good Housekeeping.* "Passport Fashions."

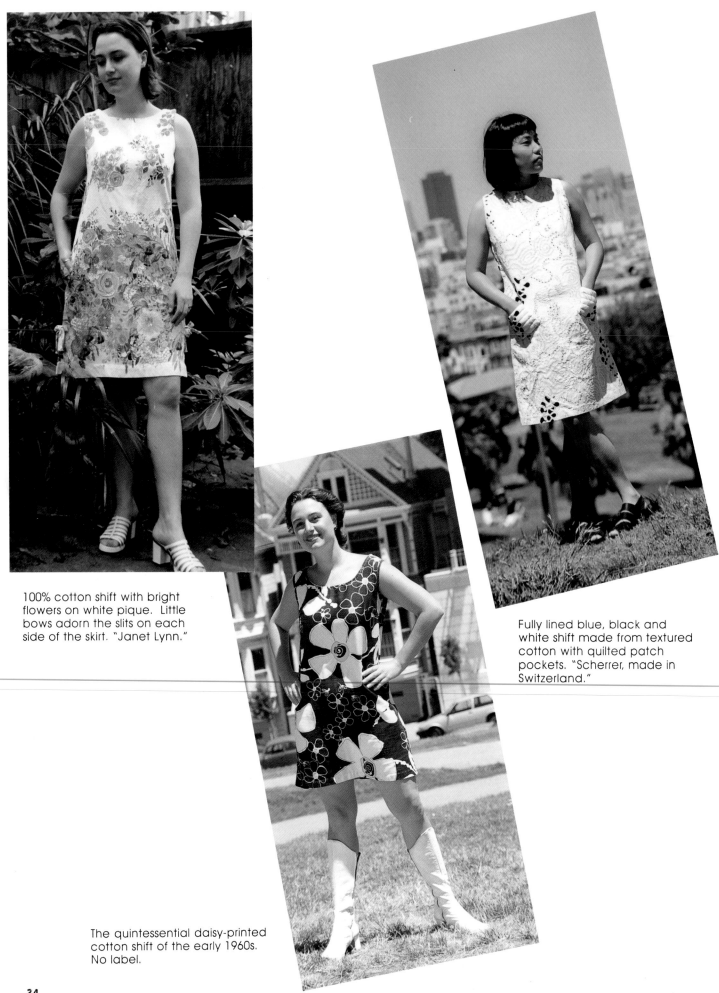

100% cotton shift with bright flowers on white pique. Little bows adorn the slits on each side of the skirt. "Janet Lynn."

Fully lined blue, black and white shift made from textured cotton with quilted patch pockets. "Scherrer, made in Switzerland."

The quintessential daisy-printed cotton shift of the early 1960s. No label.

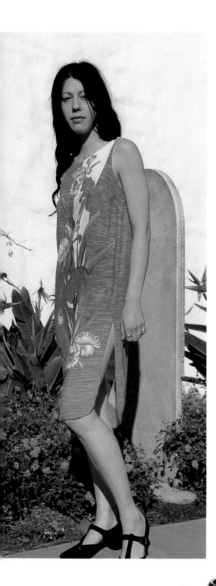

Cotton shift with a high slit up the side. "Kuonakakai authentic Hawaiian originals."

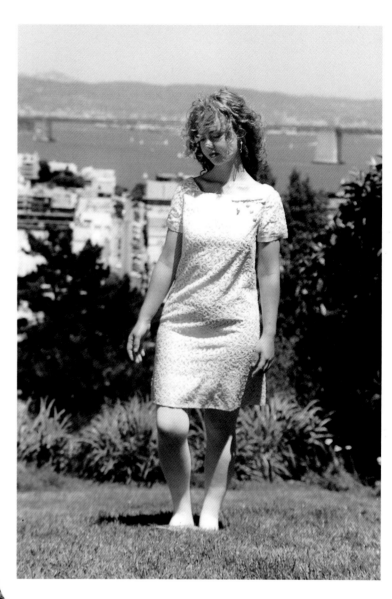

Beige lace shift is fully lined in yellow, and although the label is long gone, the exquisite hand stitching on the lining leads me to believe that it's from some designer's boutique.

100% polyester jersey brown print shift. "Collector's Items by Anne Fogarty." Matching hat is all orange feathers.

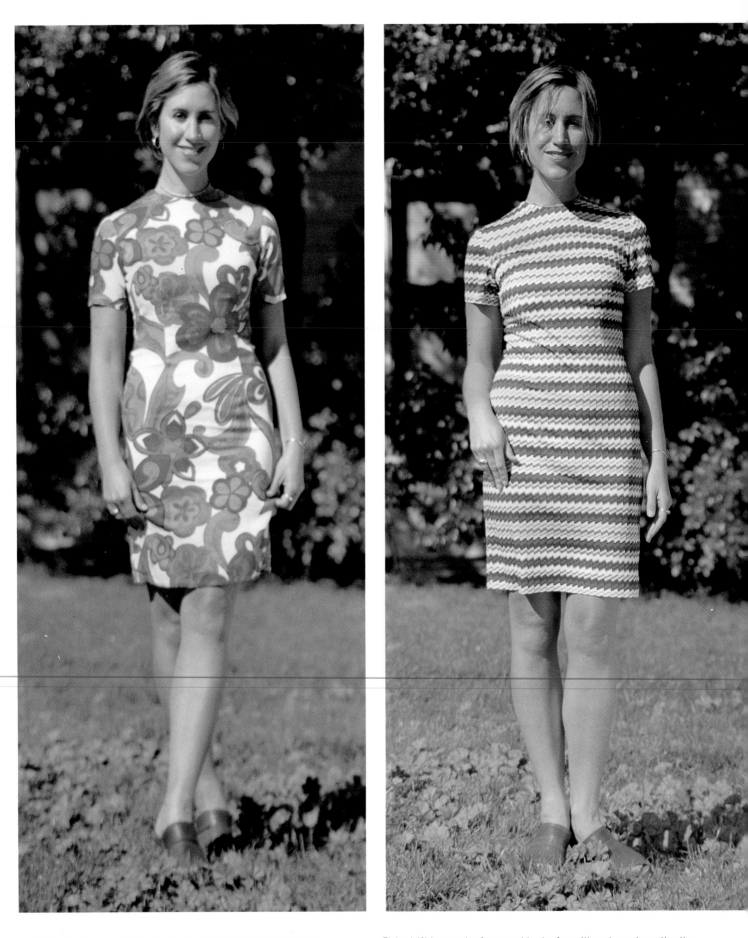

Polyester jersey shift printed with bright flowers and paisleys on white.

This shift is made from a kind of multi-colored synthetic stretch lace.

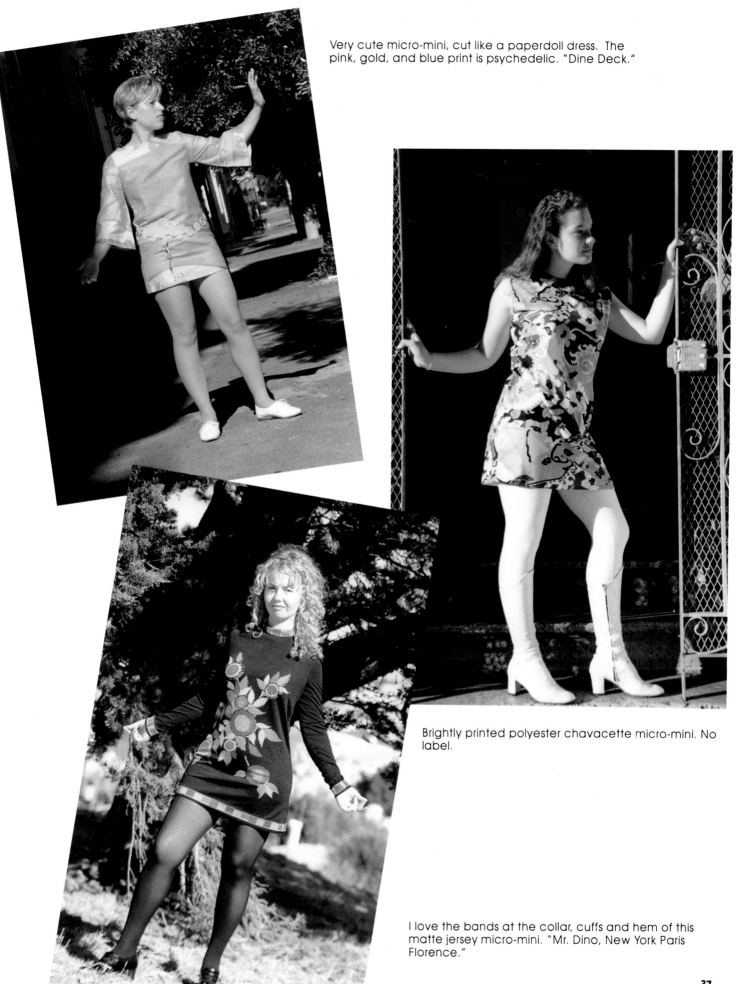

Very cute micro-mini, cut like a paperdoll dress. The pink, gold, and blue print is psychedelic. "Dine Deck."

Brightly printed polyester chavacette micro-mini. No label.

I love the bands at the collar, cuffs and hem of this matte jersey micro-mini. "Mr. Dino, New York Paris Florence."

Knit micro-mini has silver threads among the creme, rhinestone buttons and an elaborate cord trim. The label reads, "Designed Exclusively by Cabot" and tells us it's made from 52% linen, 33% Arnel triacetate, and 15% metallic yarn.

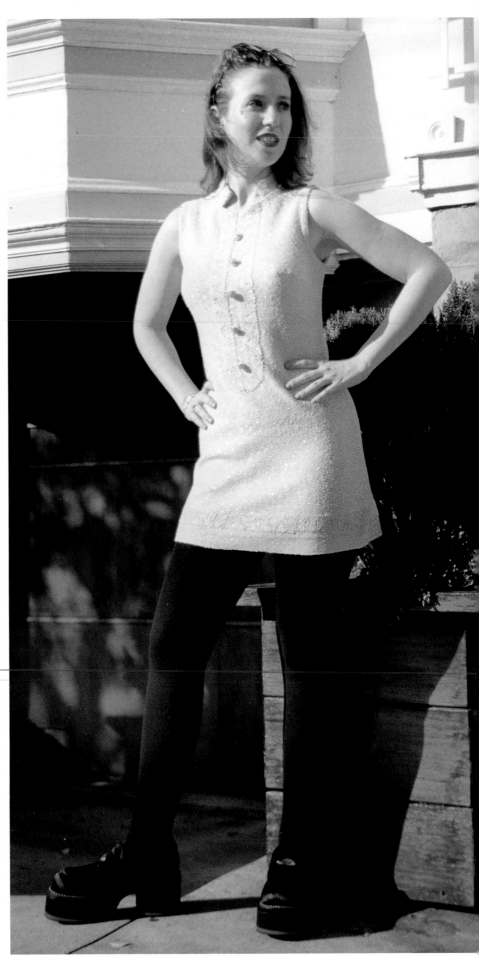

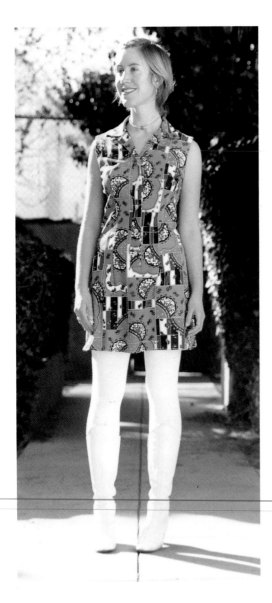

A nice little sleeveless polyester shift, printed in blue, lavender and green paisley pattern. "McInerny, Hawaii."

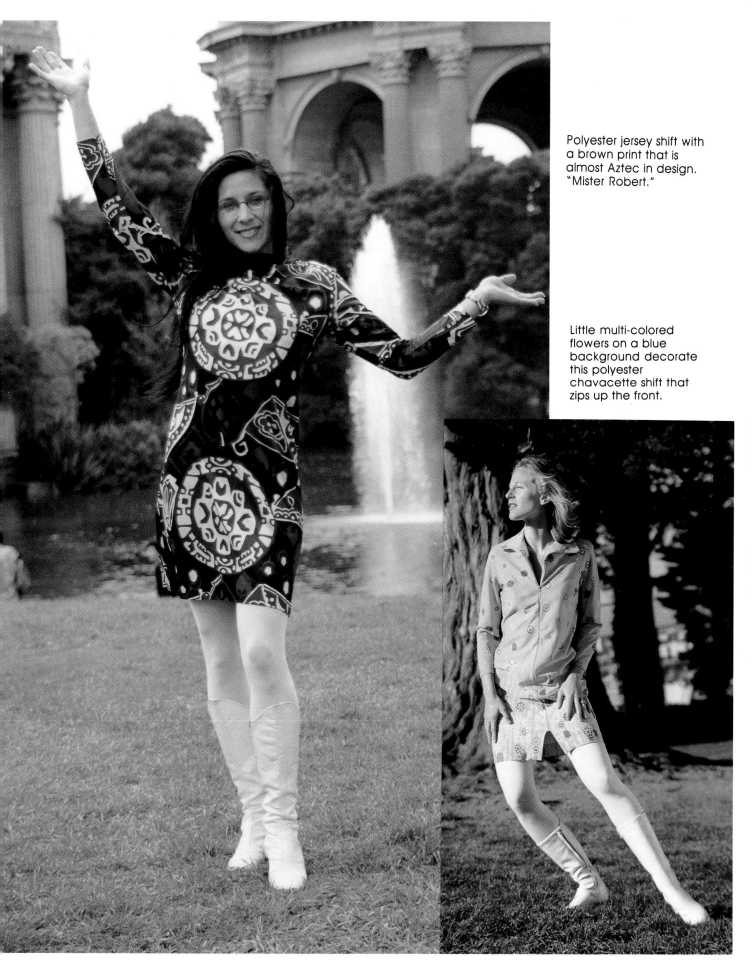

Polyester jersey shift with a brown print that is almost Aztec in design. "Mister Robert."

Little multi-colored flowers on a blue background decorate this polyester chavacette shift that zips up the front.

39

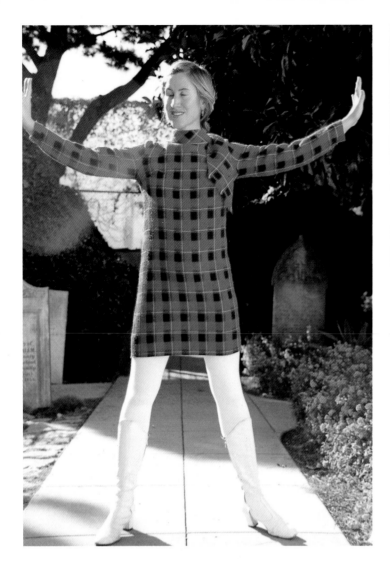

Lovely red and black plaid shift, probably wool. The scarf ends of the high collar pass through a loop at the left shoulder, so that one end emerges in front, the other in back. No label.

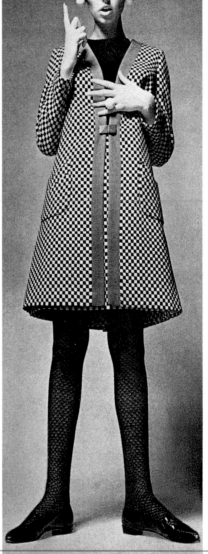

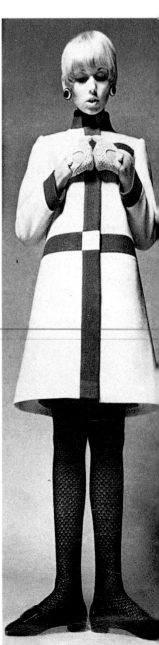

The A-Line

When the basic shift widened from the armholes through the hips to the hem, it became an A-line dress. *Look* magazine for April 5, 1966, heralded the arrival of the A-line with these words:

"After seeing what youth hath wrought in the stylish silhouette — little-girl dresses floating inches above the knee and pants suits copied from little boys' — grownups may well wonder what in the world of fickle fashion they are in for. This Spring there is hope for the aged (over 19) and affluent. Norman Norell, America's high priest of prestige dressing, has created a young look for women (those able to pay from $400 to $2,000 for a design) by adapting the A-line popular in Paris in the '50s." Needless to say, the ink was hardly dry on this article when prices of A-line dresses dropped to the level of what the average American woman could afford.

A-line dresses from *Look*, April 15, 1966.

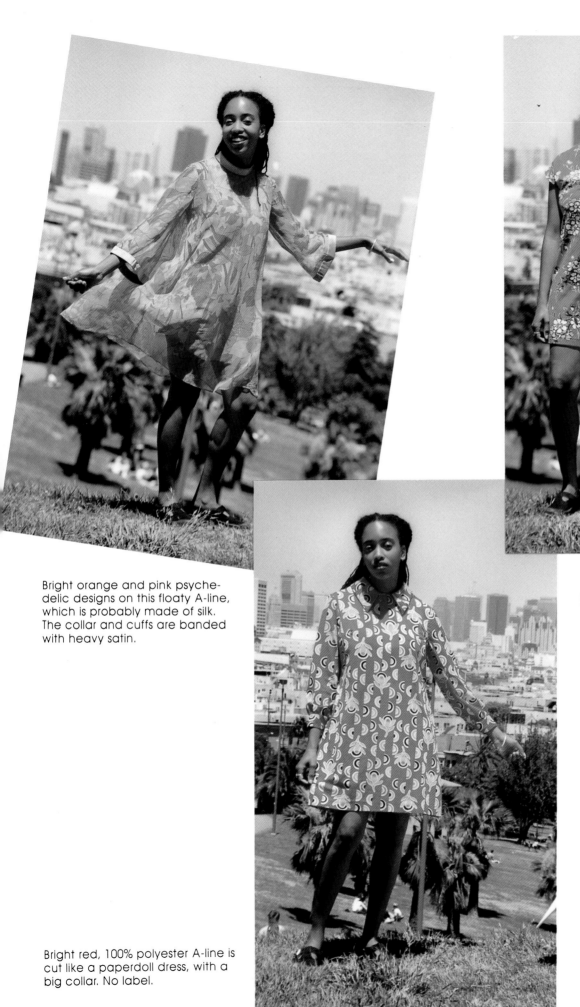

Bright orange and pink psychedelic designs on this floaty A-line,
which is probably made of silk.
The collar and cuffs are banded
with heavy satin.

Bright red polyester
jersey A-line. The only
label says, "American
Rag Compagnie,
California, U.S.A.",
which is the name of a
contemporary high-end
vintage store in San
Francisco.

Bright red, 100% polyester A-line is
cut like a paperdoll dress, with a
big collar. No label.

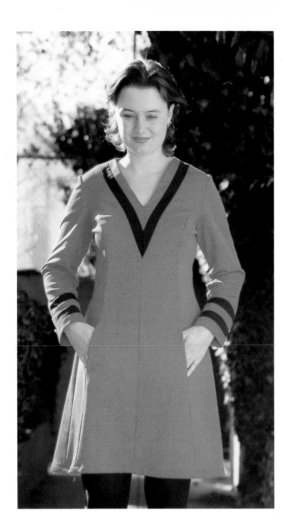

This proper little pink A-line is reminiscent of Jackie Kennedy's prim look. A pink grosgrain ribbon, matching the collar, runs down the front with embroidered scallops on either side. It's 100% rayon, and it's a "Carol Brent."

Bright red, double-knit polyester A-line looks like a costume from *Star Trek*. "Wallachs."

This is the most "Little Orphan Annie" dress I've ever seen, outside of the comic strip! Bright coral double-knit polyester with matching checked fabric at the collar, cuffs, and patch pockets.

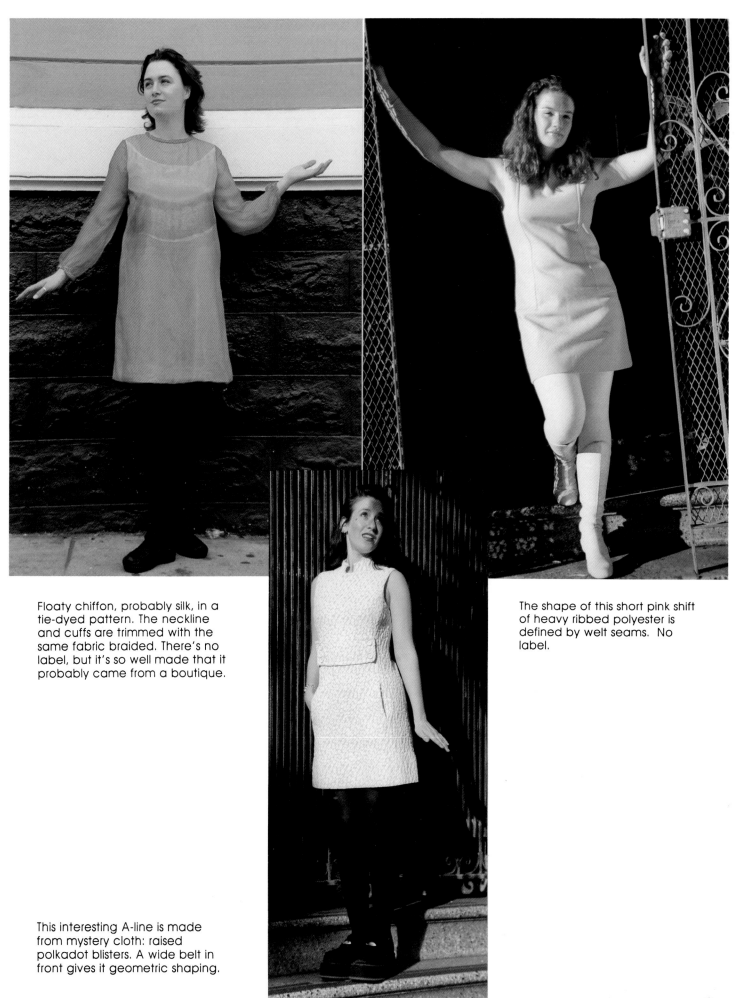

Floaty chiffon, probably silk, in a tie-dyed pattern. The neckline and cuffs are trimmed with the same fabric braided. There's no label, but it's so well made that it probably came from a boutique.

The shape of this short pink shift of heavy ribbed polyester is defined by welt seams. No label.

This interesting A-line is made from mystery cloth: raised polkadot blisters. A wide belt in front gives it geometric shaping.

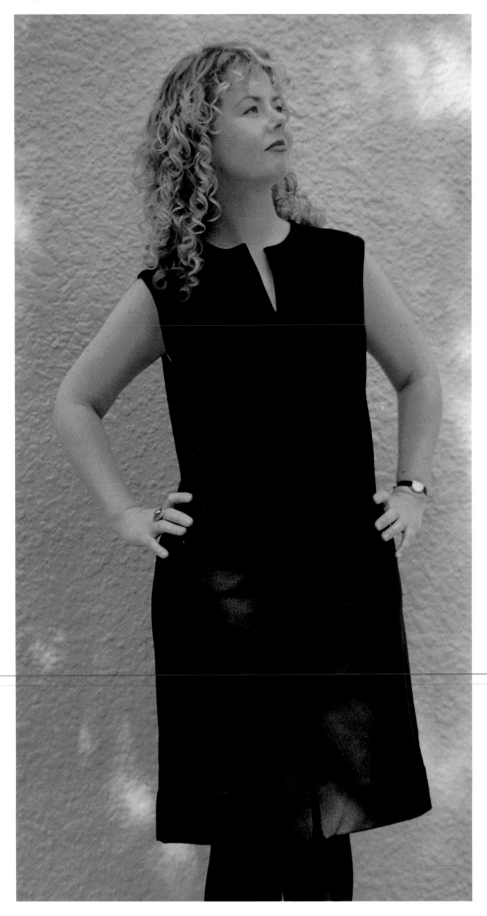

The New Geometry

Sometimes the A-line or shift was interpreted in bold solid colors like a Mondrian painting (I especially love the bright greens and oranges), made in heavy double-knit polyesters that kept their geometric shapes. These shapes were emphasized with geometric seaming. The first shifts were sleeveless garments, but when sleeves were added, they were usually kept simple and geometric. One popular way to keep a geometrically shaped dress from being boring, especially when it was cut from a solid-colored fabric, was to trim it at the collar, cuffs or hem with rows of beading or fancy braid trim.

Turquoise, double-knit A-line has geometric seaming at the waist. "Jersey House."

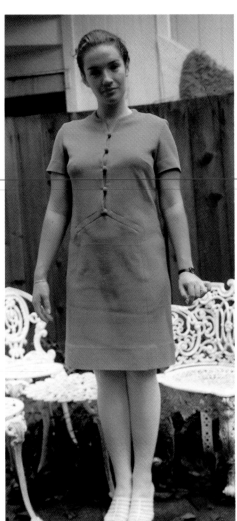

You have to look closely at this black double-knit shift to see the row of diamond-shaped seams at the waist. "Koret of Philadelphia."

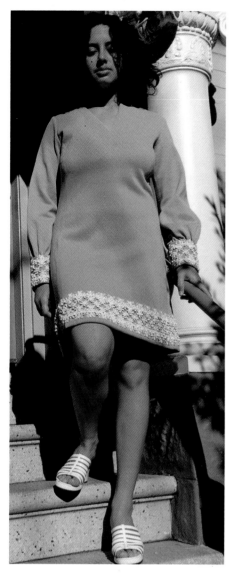

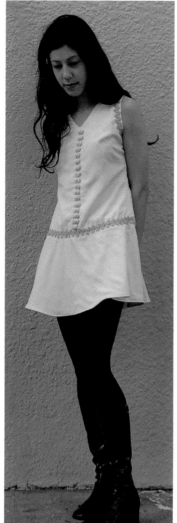

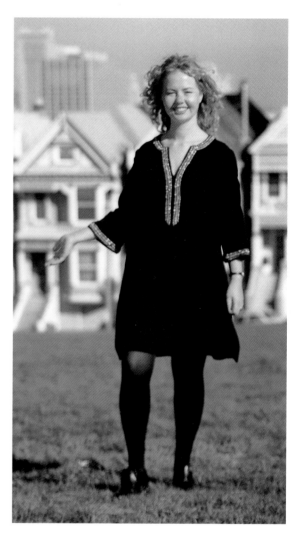

Pale yellow, linen-weave A-line with a row of self-covered buttons down the front and glittery braid at the low waist and armholes. "Delina's Quezon City."

Blue double-knit, wool A-line trimmed with heavy white beads at the hem and cuffs. It's very well made in Hong Kong, with lots of hand-stitching, and the label reads "Imperial."

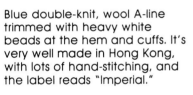

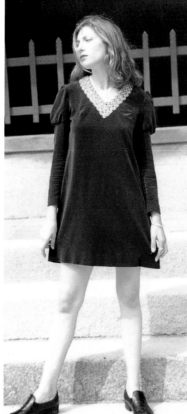

Elegant, black crepe A-line trimmed with heavy gold braid at the neckline and edges of the wide sleeves. No label, but it's fully lined and all the inside seam edges are overcast, which indicates that it comes from some chic boutique.

A wide row of gold braid trims the V-neckline of this maroon velvet A-line. The best parts are the poetic sleeves, pouffed at the top and form-fitting at the wrist. No label.

Chapter Four
The Granny Dress

Long, flowered dresses originated in California and the French Riviera in the early '60s, as beach or resort wear. They were quickly adopted by savvy British "birds" who wore the long dresses in London and created a fashionable alternative to mini dresses. Called "granny dresses" they were reminiscent of old-fashioned country dresses like those your "granny" might have worn. For many young Americans, they symbolized a rebellion against what they considered the sterile, plastic life of the fifties. By the later '60s, the granny dress had become the uniform for young American "hippies" who moved to communes in the country. Some granny dresses were trimmed with bright beads, macramé or heavy cotton crochet for a hand-crafted look. Not surprisingly, during this period many women took up the art of handmade crochet and macramé.

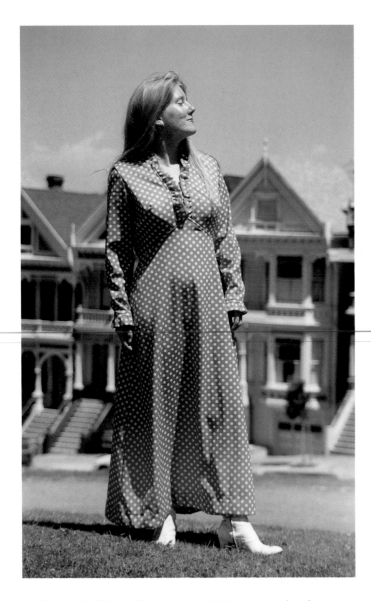

Ruffles and white polkadots on bright green polyester jersey. No label.

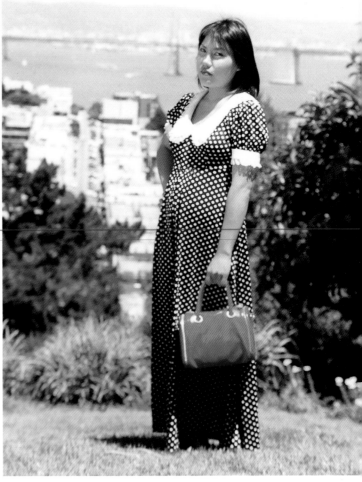

White, lace-trimmed collar and cuffs and white polkadots on navy blue polyester jersey. No label.

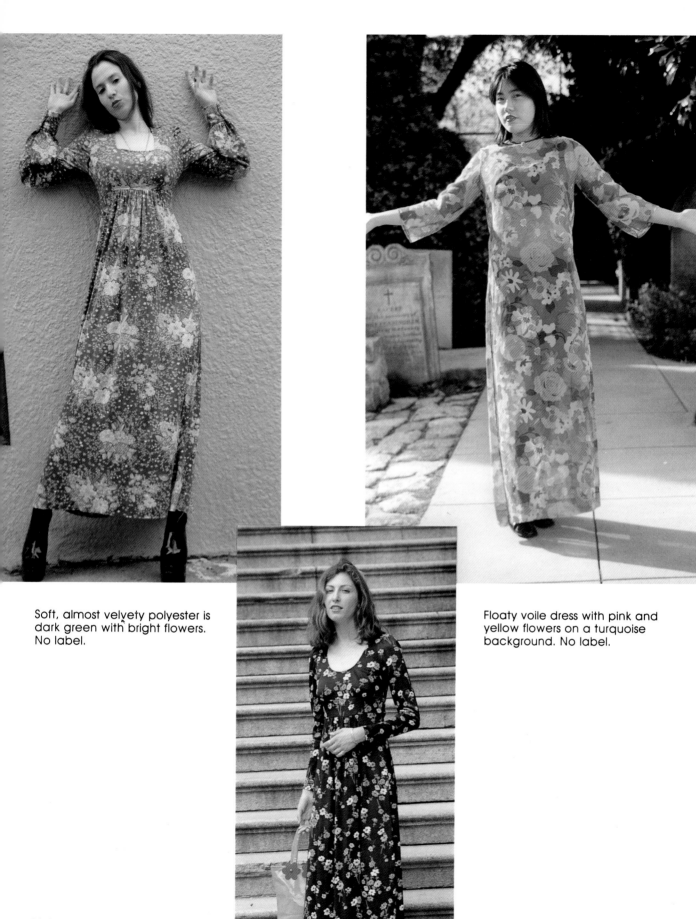

Soft, almost velvety polyester is dark green with bright flowers. No label.

Floaty voile dress with pink and yellow flowers on a turquoise background. No label.

Multi-colored posies on dark green, 100% triacetate. The high waisted dress ties in back, and the label reads "Phase II, California."

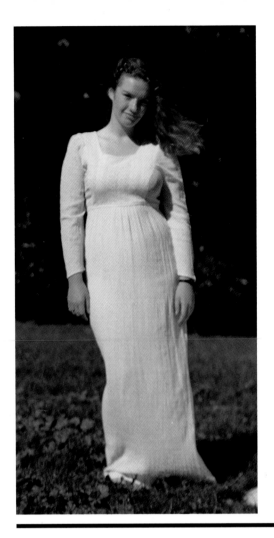

The bodice of this long cotton gauze dress is heavy lace, and it ties in the back. The only part of the label that's left says it's made in India.

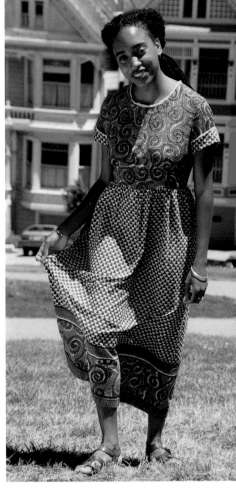

Long African-print cotton dress is trimmed at the neckline and cuffs with crocheted lace. The label reads "Raymodes" and Abra says it reminds her of an African Laura Ashley.

Patchwork

Granny dresses from the early '60s featured calico and patchwork prints (like on quilts) although, ironically, sometimes the patchwork was printed on polyester! The use of patchwork, like the granny dress, represented a return to simpler times and was compatible with the youth's preference for organic foods (whether from an actual preference or monetary need is not important here) and appeared in every conceivable way, on every conceivable outfit.

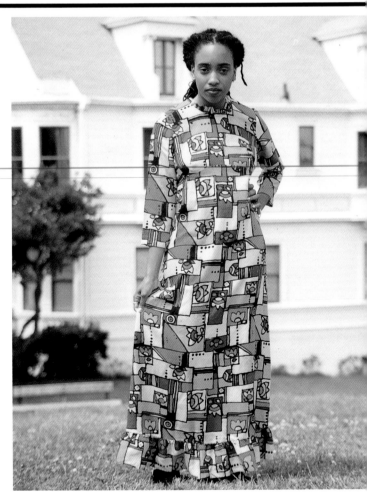

Acrylic granny dress in a psychedelic patchwork print of orange, gold and tan earthtones. Ruffles at the hem and neckline, and the label reads "Charlotta of California, by Glazier."

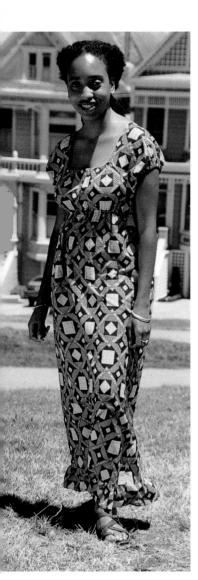

Very flattering empire patchwork print granny with a ruffle at
the hem. No label.

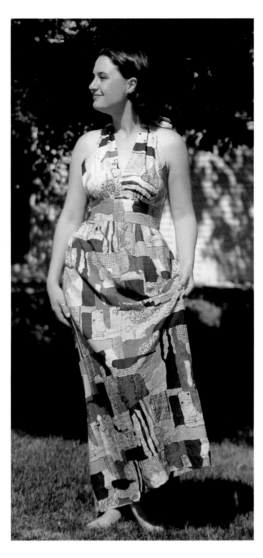

Cotton halter-necked sundress
in a multi-colored patchwork
print. "Mr.'B' of California."

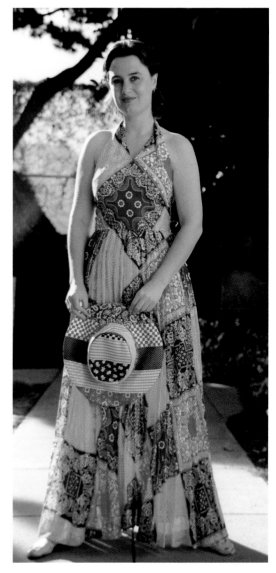

Patchwork bandanna print
sundress has a halter neck and
is made from voile, and fully
lined with more voile. The long
skirt is permanently pleated.

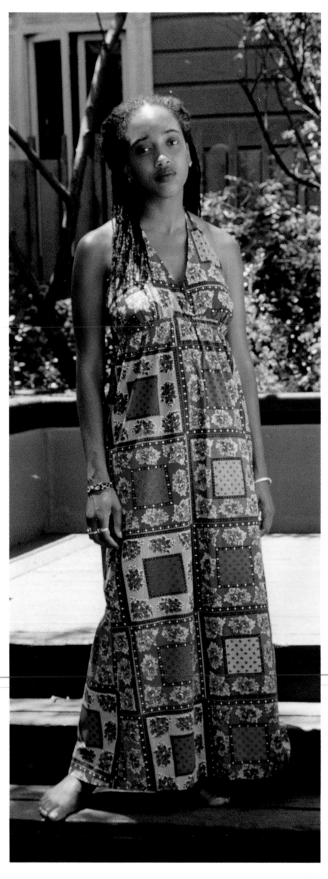

Front and side views of a favorite cotton patchwork print halter dress. "Fritzi."

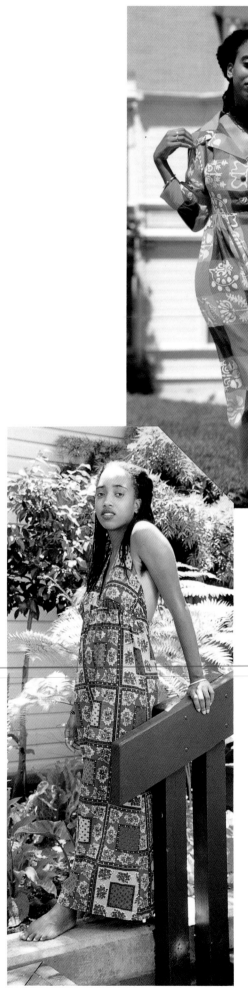

This graceful patchwork print dress is fully lined, except for the sleeves. The filmy fabric is probably silk organza, but there's no label to tell us.

Brown and white, patchwork print bathing suit would serve nicely as a playsuit today. "Carol & Mary by Nalii, Honolulu."

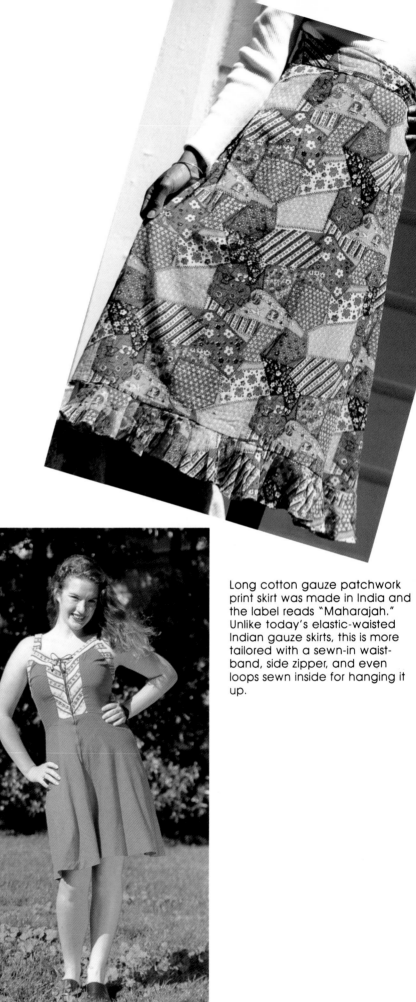

Long cotton gauze patchwork print skirt was made in India and the label reads "Maharajah." Unlike today's elastic-waisted Indian gauze skirts, this is more tailored with a sewn-in waistband, side zipper, and even loops sewn inside for hanging it up.

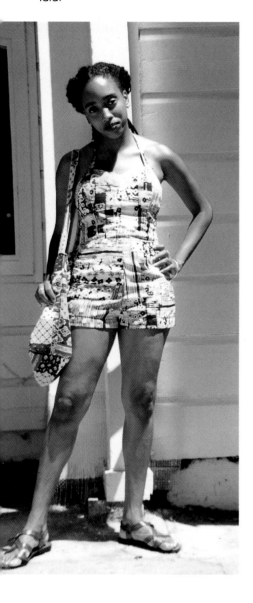

Country-girl, rust-colored, cotton sundress trimmed with woven striped material that looks Guatemalan, and tied in front with a rust-colored cord that ends in bright wooden beads.

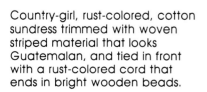

51

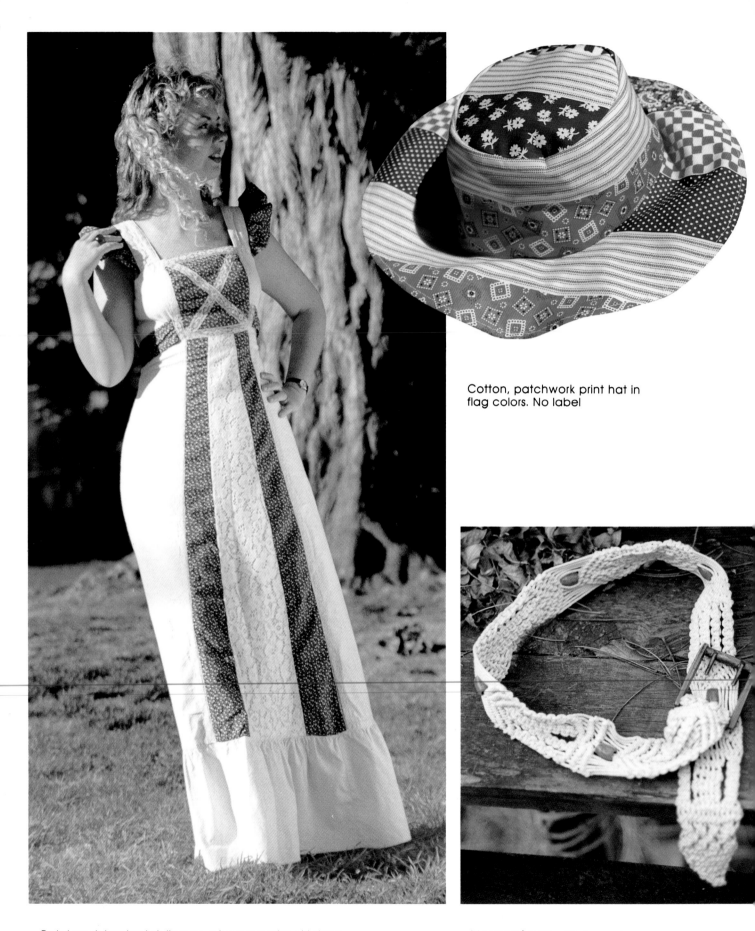

Cotton, patchwork print hat in flag colors. No label

Patchwork-inspired styling on a long country-girl dress. It's made from a combination of muslin, calico, and two kinds of lace.

Macramé belt with turquoise beads woven into the strands.

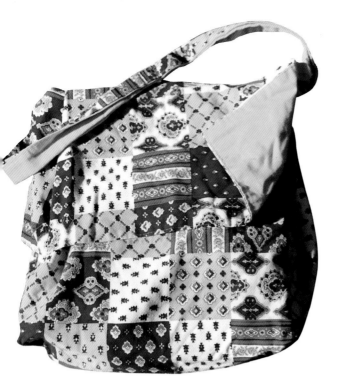

Cotton patchwork print shoulder-bag lined in yellow cotton.

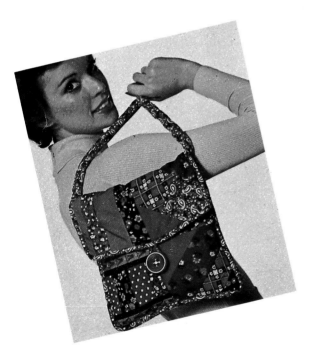

A do-it-yourself patchwork shoulder-bag from *Woman's Day*, May, 1974.

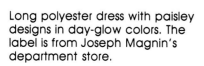

Long polyester dress with paisley designs in day-glow colors. The label is from Joseph Magnin's department store.

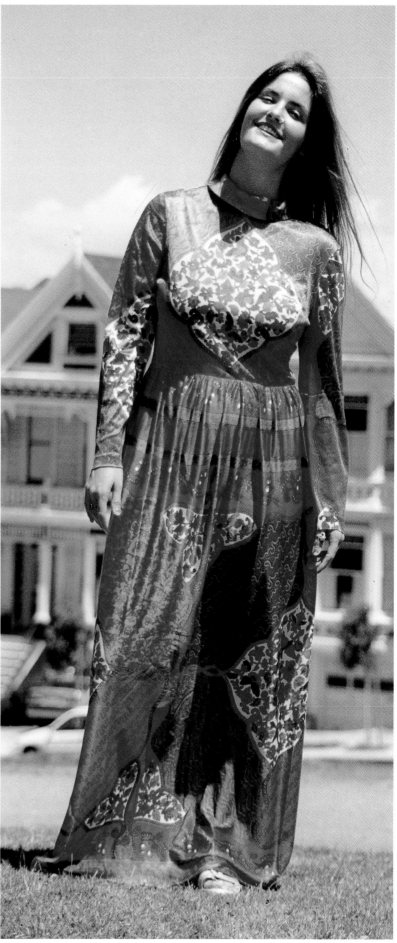

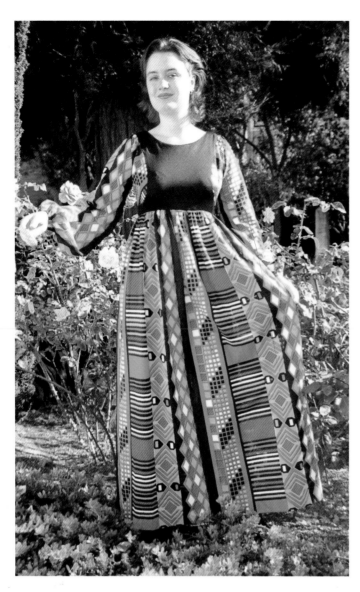

Long dress made from a polyester woven like terrycloth and velvet. The print is a mind-boggling, eye-popping combination of stripes, windowpanes, and diamonds in red, green, yellow, and blue!

Fully lined, long polyester dress with a keyhole cut-out at the neckline. No label.

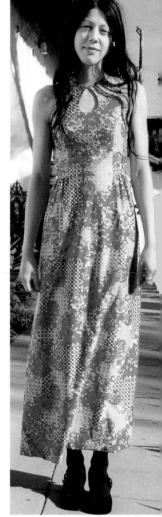

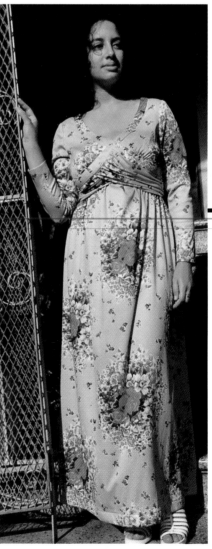

Granny Gets "Hip"

By the late 1960s, the long dress which had originally been intended as a simple, homey style became a sophisticated long dress to be worn by society women at cocktail parties. Fabrics were now unabashed polyesters, prints grew more abstract and psychedelic, and the hitherto old-fashioned styling grew positively vampy, with deep necklines or high side slits in the skirts. Of course, the country-style granny didn't go away; old-fashioned, organic-looking long dresses continued to be worn through the '70s.

Very graceful, long, 100% polyester dress with draped bodice. "Henry-Lee."

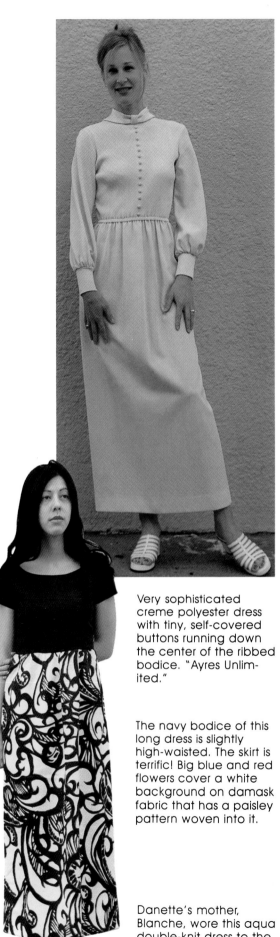

Very sophisticated creme polyester dress with tiny, self-covered buttons running down the center of the ribbed bodice. "Ayres Unlimited."

The navy bodice of this long dress is slightly high-waisted. The skirt is terrific! Big blue and red flowers cover a white background on damask fabric that has a paisley pattern woven into it.

Danette's mother, Blanche, wore this aqua double-knit dress to the wedding of her sister, Charlene, in 1968.

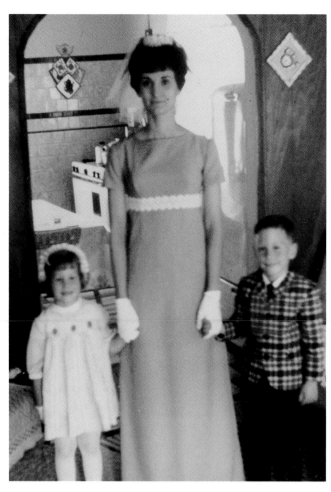

Here's Blanche, wearing the aqua dress, as seen on page 55, to her sister's wedding in 1968.

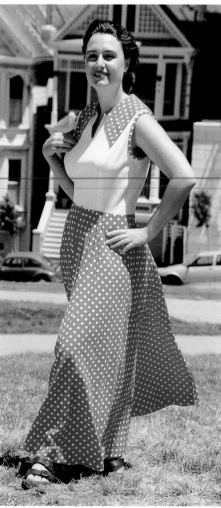

The polkadot skirt of this long "Minnie Mouse" dress is permanently pleated. "Donovan Galvani of Dallas."

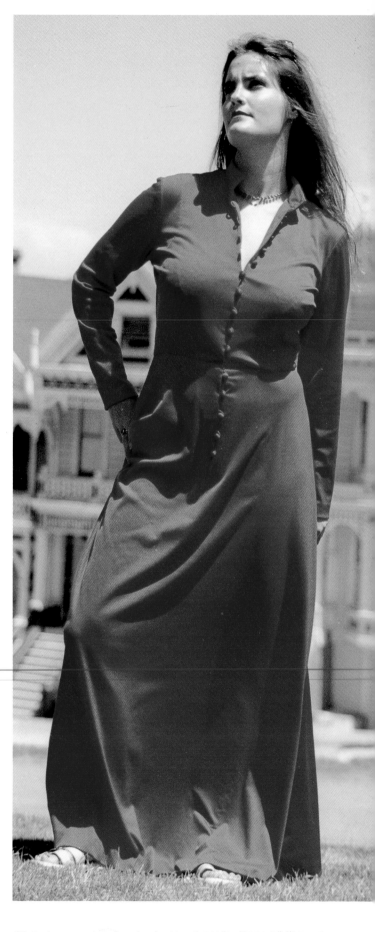

Slinky long red polyester jersey dress buttons all the way up the front with little self-covered buttons and button loops. "Tori Richards for I. Magnin and Co., Honolulu."

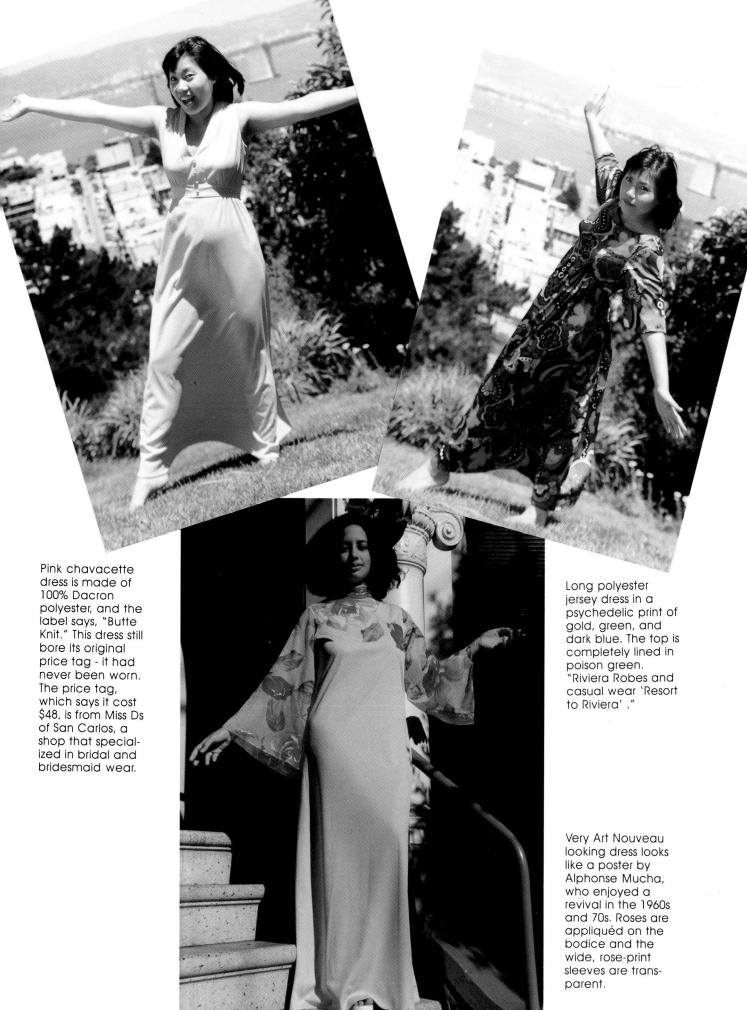

Pink chavacette dress is made of 100% Dacron polyester, and the label says, "Butte Knit." This dress still bore its original price tag - it had never been worn. The price tag, which says it cost $48, is from Miss Ds of San Carlos, a shop that specialized in bridal and bridesmaid wear.

Long polyester jersey dress in a psychedelic print of gold, green, and dark blue. The top is completely lined in poison green. "Riviera Robes and casual wear 'Resort to Riviera' ."

Very Art Nouveau looking dress looks like a poster by Alphonse Mucha, who enjoyed a revival in the 1960s and 70s. Roses are appliquéd on the bodice and the wide, rose-print sleeves are transparent.

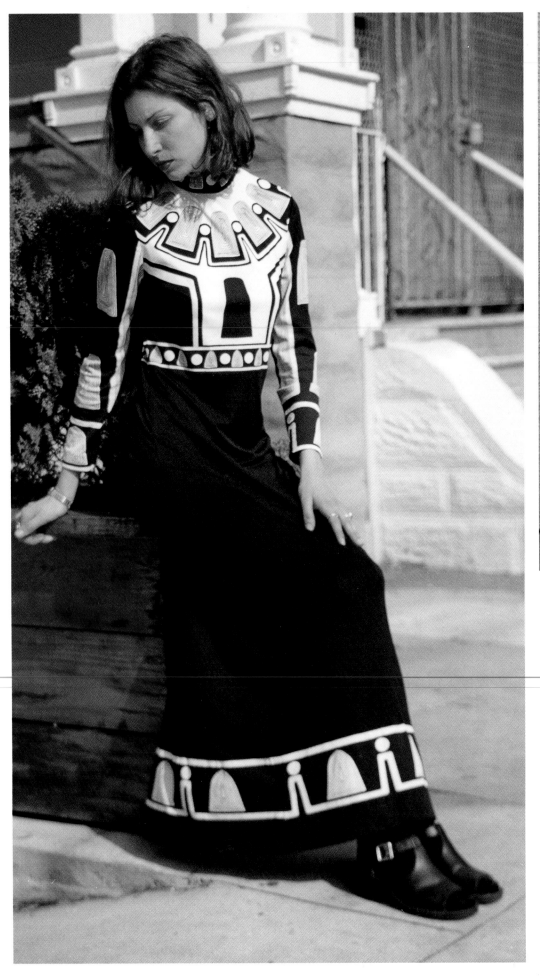

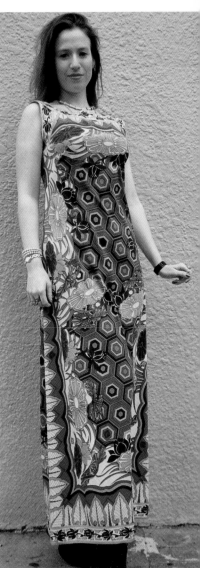

This Egyptian looking dress is beautifully constructed inside, and was probably very expensive. The label says, "Made in Italy for Holt Renfrew."

Another Egyptian looking dress, this one in a black and white print on matte jersey, very sophisticated. No label.

Chapter Five

*P*aisley & The East

During this time, Beatle musician George Harrison played the sitar, and the Beatles went to India to study with their own guru.

India was found to be in the forefront of fashion. Young men of fashion wore Nehru jackets and everybody meditated. The April, 1965 issue of *Vogue* devoted most of its space to something they called "Scheherazaderie" featuring models in bizarre get-ups from some Arabian nightmare. They got positively poetic about it, too: "...it's new again in this year's fashion...the lure of Eastern seraglios and Arab nights...gauzy chemises, fluent robes, and chalwar trousers...Kohl around the eyes, the undiluted scents of rose, patchouli, ambergris, and musk...with all the indolent grace of Turquerie to charm the sheik at home."

The average woman was content to wear clothing with distinctive "paisley" (scrolled leaf) motifs and scent herself with patchouli (an Indian mint with an oil of distinctive scent). The scrolled leaf design motifs and patchouli fragrance go way back together; the relationship started in the first half of the nineteenth century when exquisite and very expensive woven "cashmere" shawls with a colorful scrolled leaf motif that were imported from Kashmir, India, were all the rage. Owning one of these shawls was very much the equivalent of owning a mink coat today. When shipped to Europe and America, the shawls would be packed in dried patchouli flowers, which are a natural moth repellent, so they arrived smelling like patchouli. Thus, the smell of patchouli was associated with expensive cashmere shawls, and by scenting themselves with patchouli oil, women who couldn't afford to wear the shawls could at least smell like they did. By the mid-nineteeth century, factories in Paisley, Scotland, started manufacturing less expensive copies of the "cashmere" shawls and the name "paisley" became the popular name for the new shawls with the scrolled leaf motif. As always happens, once everybody could afford one, both "cashmere" and "Paisley" shawls quickly went out of style, as did the scent associated with them. When the popularity of the paisley motif was revived in the 1960s, patchouli once more came along, and soon all the chic young things smelled like Indian insect repellent. (I'm being a bit unfair here; it so happens that I still wear patchouli, and love it!)

Clothing made in India arrived in America towards the end of the 1960s as an exotic trickle and grew to a tidal

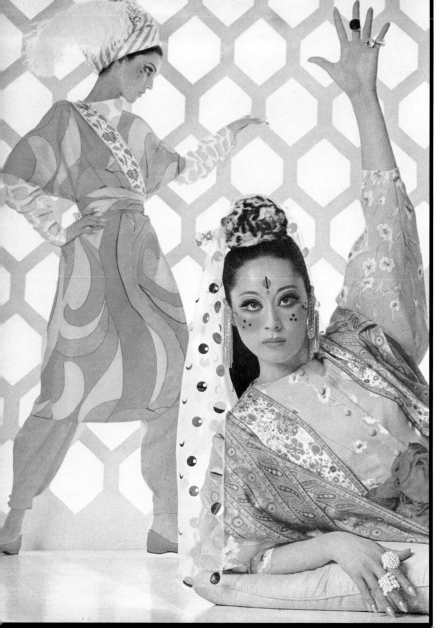

Illustration from *Vogue*, April 1965, for their article,"Scheherazaderie."

wave by the '70s. Inexpensive, gauzy imports in both yardgoods and finished clothing were exciting to young Americans who decorated their rooms with Indian bedspreads and tacked mandalas on their walls. Today, Indian imports are still with us, but we've grown used to them, and we no longer rhapsodize over a label that says "Made in India." (Prediction: 25 years from now, all those gauzy rayon tiered skirts from the early '90s will be avidly collected!)

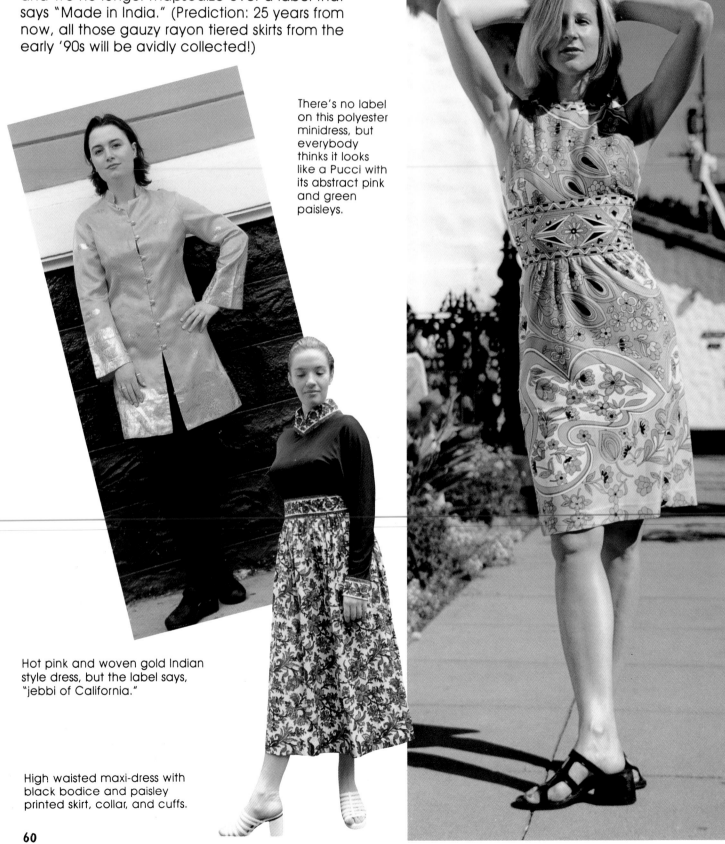

There's no label on this polyester minidress, but everybody thinks it looks like a Pucci with its abstract pink and green paisleys.

Hot pink and woven gold Indian style dress, but the label says, "jebbi of California."

High waisted maxi-dress with black bodice and paisley printed skirt, collar, and cuffs.

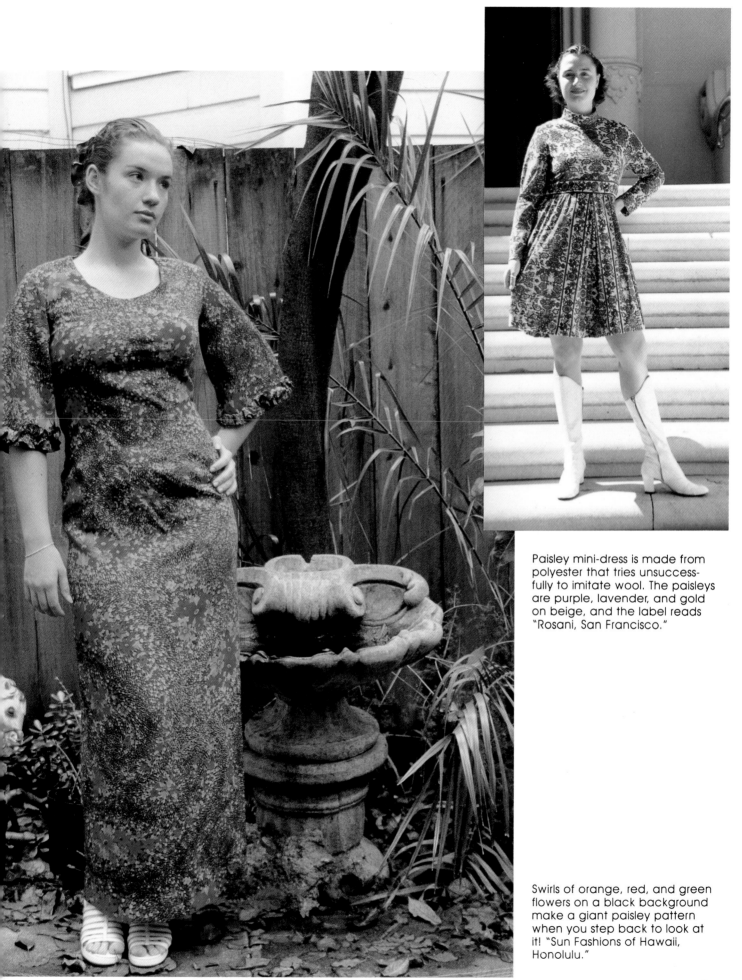

Paisley mini-dress is made from polyester that tries unsuccessfully to imitate wool. The paisleys are purple, lavender, and gold on beige, and the label reads "Rosani, San Francisco."

Swirls of orange, red, and green flowers on a black background make a giant paisley pattern when you step back to look at it! "Sun Fashions of Hawaii, Honolulu."

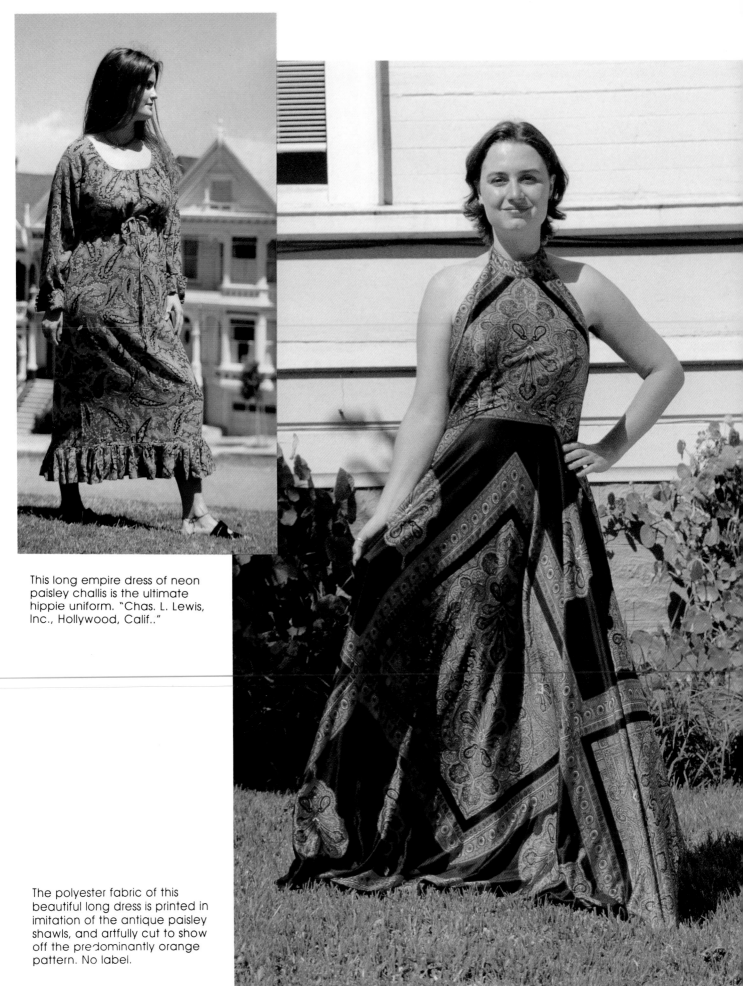

This long empire dress of neon paisley challis is the ultimate hippie uniform. "Chas. L. Lewis, Inc., Hollywood, Calif.."

The polyester fabric of this beautiful long dress is printed in imitation of the antique paisley shawls, and artfully cut to show off the predominantly orange pattern. No label.

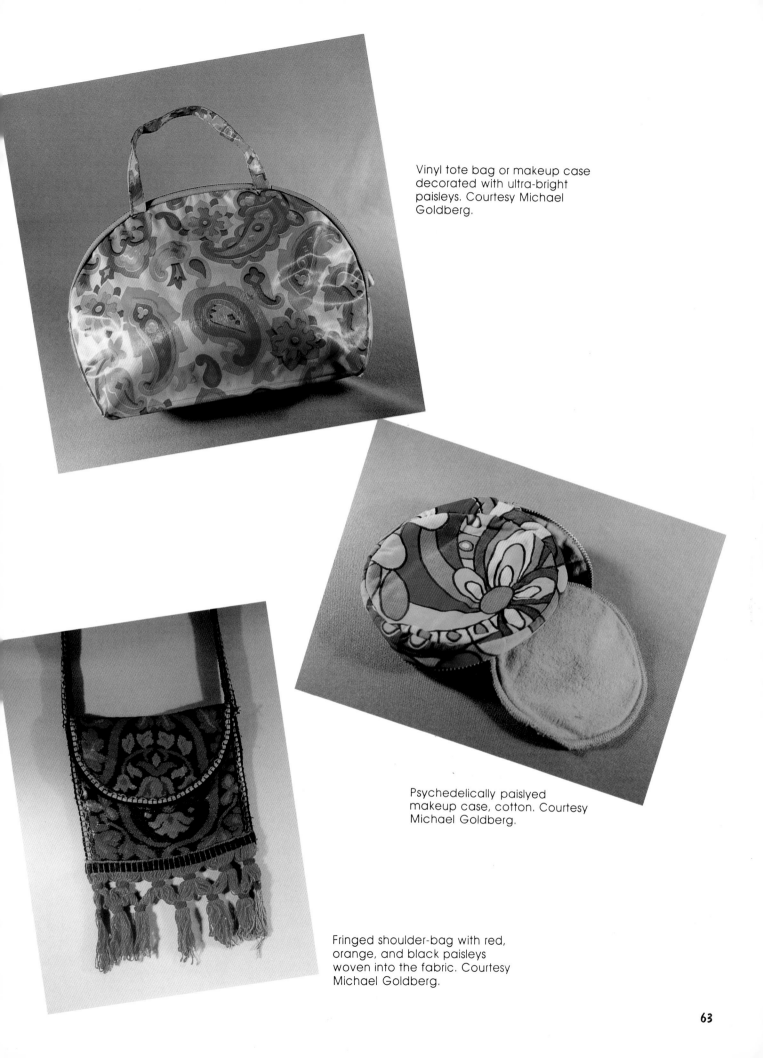

Vinyl tote bag or makeup case decorated with ultra-bright paisleys. Courtesy Michael Goldberg.

Psychedelically paislyed makeup case, cotton. Courtesy Michael Goldberg.

Fringed shoulder-bag with red, orange, and black paisleys woven into the fabric. Courtesy Michael Goldberg.

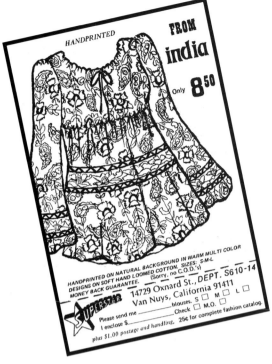

Advertisement for a blouse
imported from India, from
Seventeen, October, 1976.

Green crushed
velvet empire dress
with heavily embroi-
dered bodice,
cuffs, and hem,
made in Pakistan
for "Boluchi."

Maroon gauze blouse with
crocheted yoke and wide
angel sleeves, made in Pakistan
for "Bila."

Wraparound skirt made of batik
from Maylasia.

64

Chinese Influence

Though not as profound an influence as that from India, another fashion style made popular in the 1960s came from China, and its motivation was probably at least partly political. The war in Vietnam was extremely unpopular with many young Americans who found themselves sympathizing with the Vietnamese, and, by extension, with China. In 1967, an East Village boutique specialized in making and selling the Ao-Dai, the traditional Vietnamese dress. The shop was called Vietnam Protique, and the suffix "Pro" obviously stood for "protest." At any rate, a great many dresses from the period of the Vietnam war featured Chinese-style Mandarin collars.

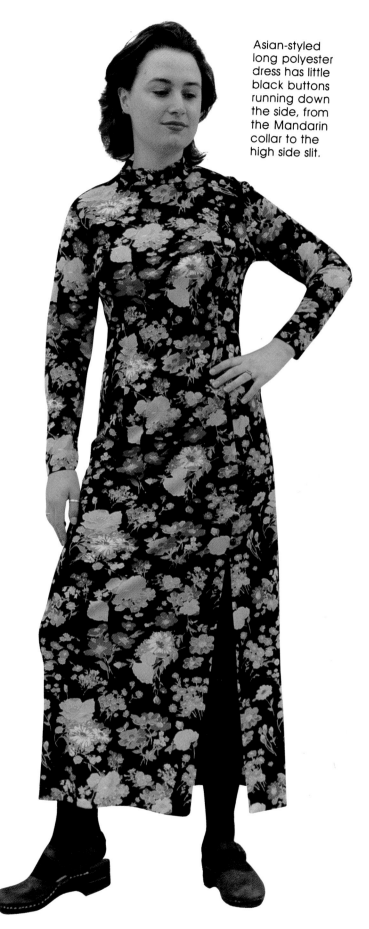

Asian-styled long polyester dress has little black buttons running down the side, from the Mandarin collar to the high side slit.

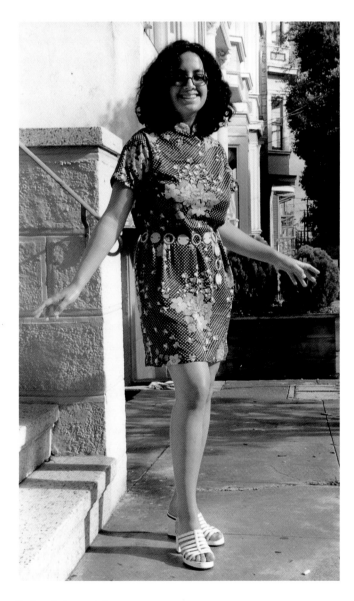

Polkadots and flowers on a polyester jersey shift with a mandarin collar.

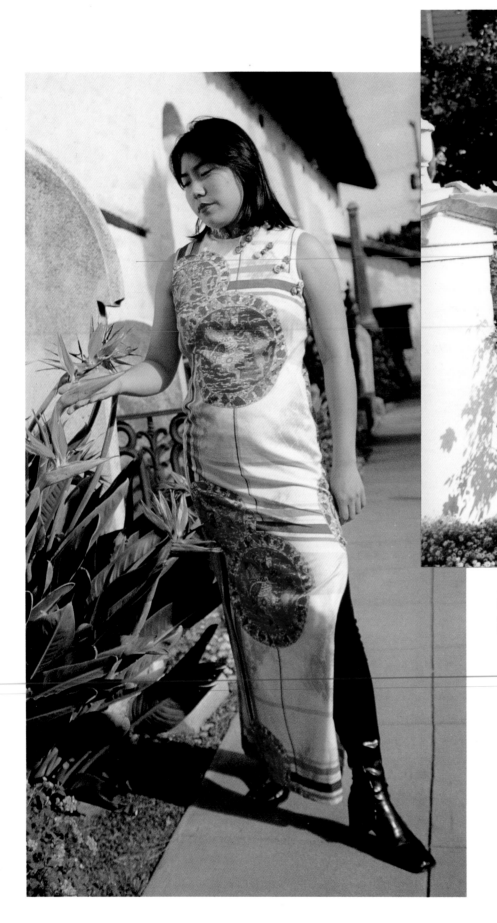

Long dress of polyester jersey has a Mandarin collar and red and yellow flowers on a black background. "It's a Lehigh."

100% cotton Chinese influenced dress has Mandarin collar, a slit at the side, and 4 frog closings. "made in Hawaii for Andrade, Honolulu."

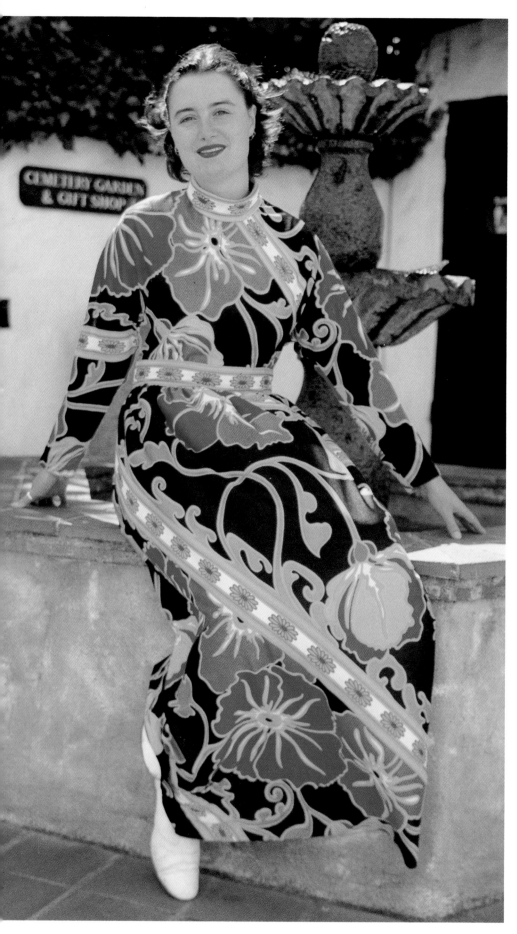

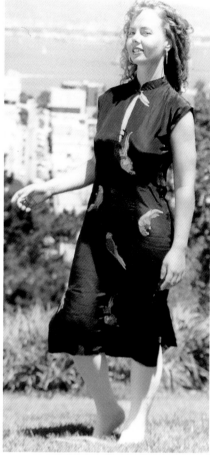

Bright parrots adorn this Chinese-inspired black 100% rayon dress, with retro styling. It actually has a side zipper, like dresses from twenty years earlier! The label says, "Moonglow, California."

Humongous red flowers adorn this long, Asian styled polyester dress. "Lori Till."

Chapter Six
Pop & Op

The 1960s in America was a time of liberal and conservative ideas that spawned warring factions about perceptions of "progress" and confidence in the state of life at that time. One faction was a movement of rebellion against the sterility of modern life, against war, and for a return to the organic, the simple and natural elements (including marijuana). Young people of this persuasion moved to communes in the country and learned organic farming. Women wore their hair long and loose and threw away their lipstick, or used such pale lipsticks that they looked like they weren't wearing any! In the cities, people went barefoot or wore sandals and they ate brown rice. In fashion, their preference was for granny dresses, patchwork prints and gingham, and the use of natural trim materials like jute and macramé. The opposing faction embraced the benefits and promises of "progress;" they gloried in science fiction and saw the movie *2001 Space Odyssey* dozens of times, loved Marvel Comics, and felt that "the future" had arrived. These peoples preferred wearing "new" garments made of paper and plastic and fabrics printed with Op (for optical) art designs and those inspired by artists like cubist Piet Mondrian, pop artist Andy Warhol, and Peter Max and some experimented with "new" halucinogens. The two factions were as different as their music: folk and heavy metal, but that didn't mean that a lot of people in the middle couldn't like them both.

She's come a long way, baby, and she wears an Op-art jacket. A Virginia Slims advertisement from *Life*, October 20, 1972.

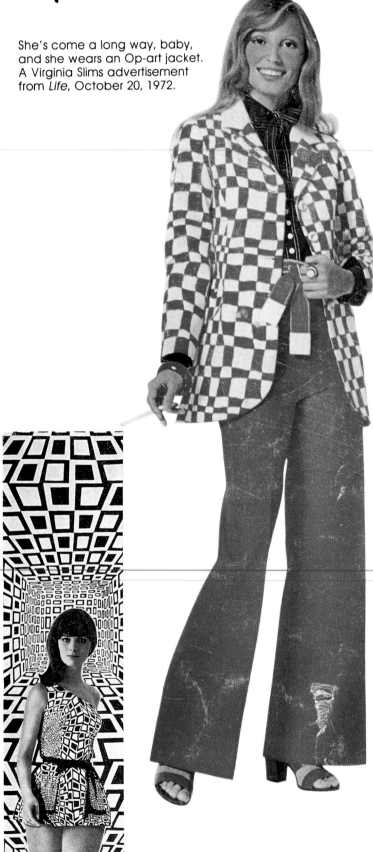

An Op-art bathing suit, from *Better Homes and Gardens*, August, 1965

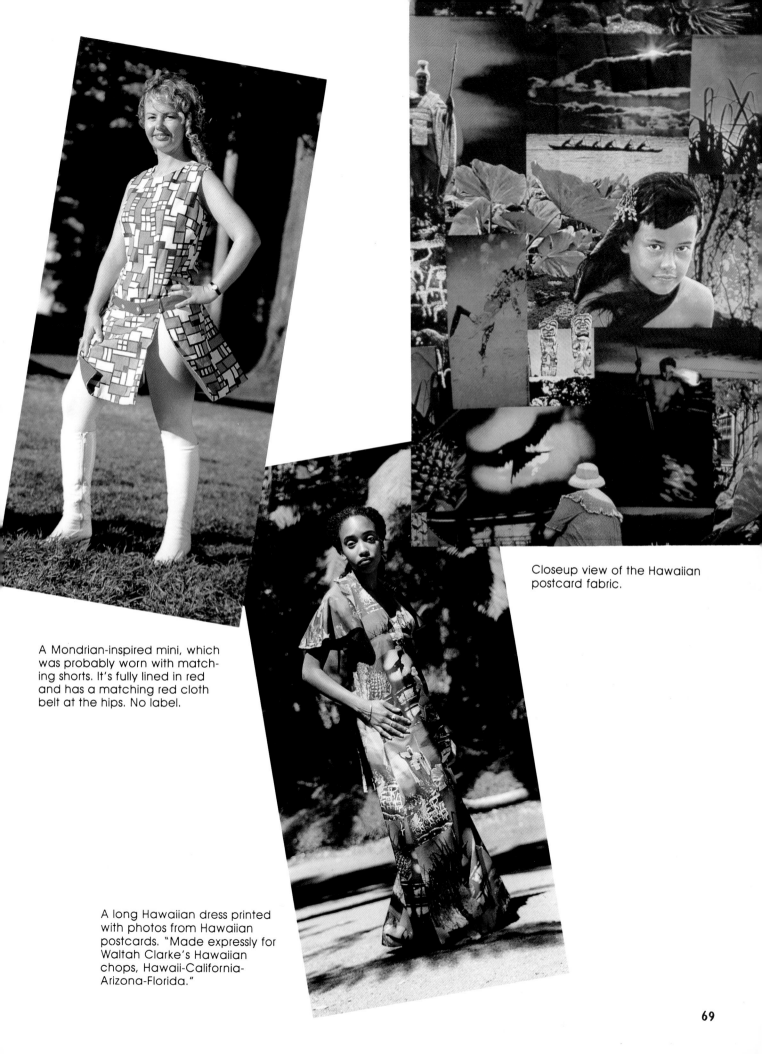

A Mondrian-inspired mini, which was probably worn with matching shorts. It's fully lined in red and has a matching red cloth belt at the hips. No label.

Closeup view of the Hawaiian postcard fabric.

A long Hawaiian dress printed with photos from Hawaiian postcards. "Made expressly for Waltah Clarke's Hawaiian chops, Hawaii-California-Arizona-Florida."

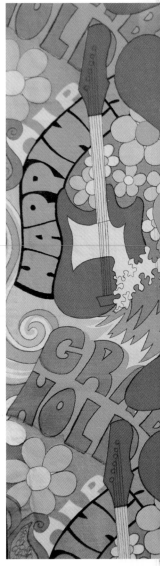

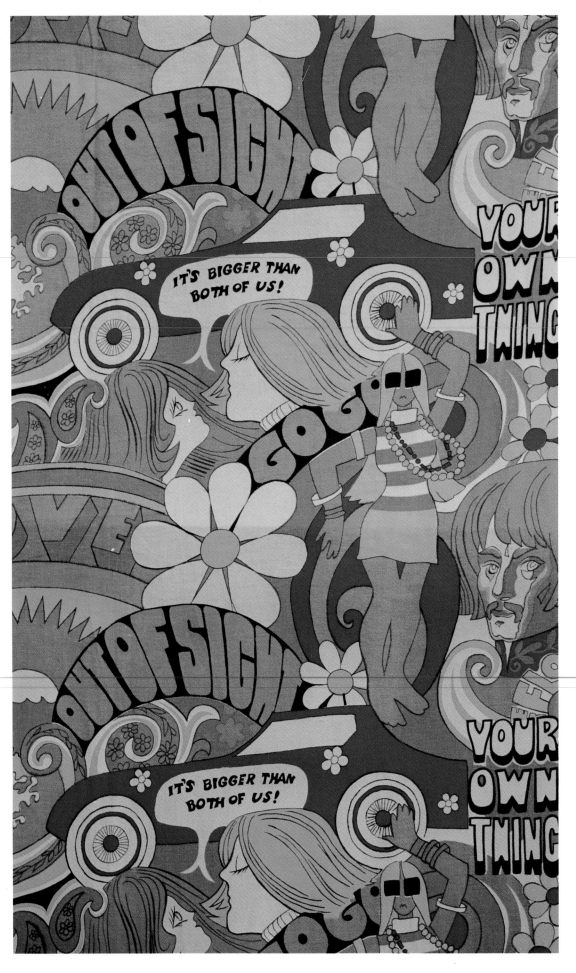

Two views of pop-art fabric featuring, among others, a dancing "chick", a surfer, and Beatle George Harrison.

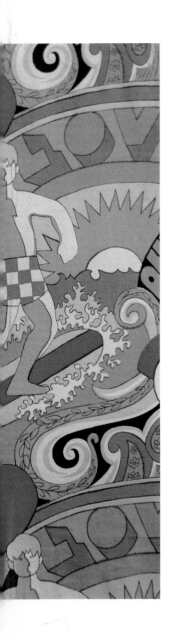

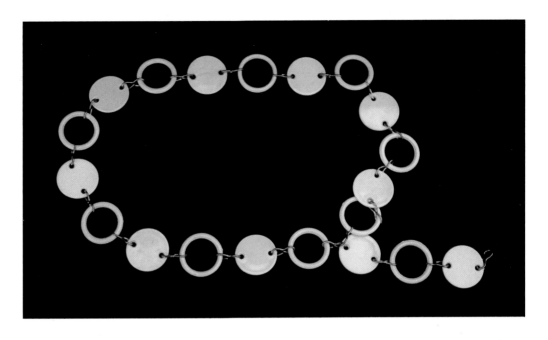

Pink plastic chain belt.

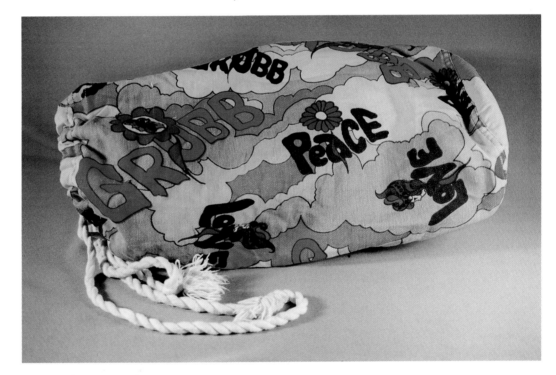

Denim tote bag with Peter Max-inspired designs. Courtesy Michael Goldberg.

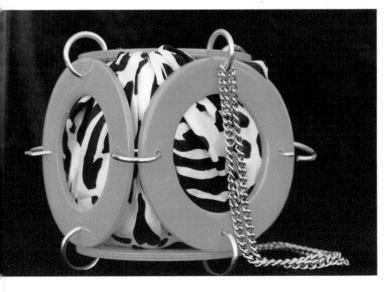

A handbag. Black and white zebra stripes, inside a cage of big orange plastic links. Courtesy Martini Mercantile.

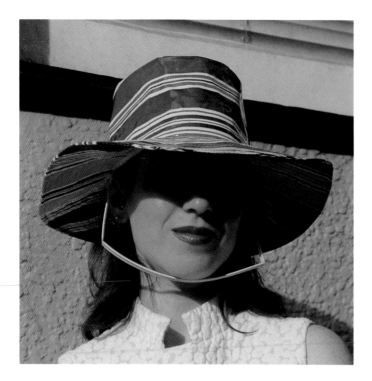

Vinyl hat with orange and green stripes.

The Flags

The '60s popular concept of wearing clothing made from an American or British flag started as a form of political protest over the war in Viet Nam. At first, young men and women were actually arrested for wearing clothes made from, or appearing to be made from, these national flags. But fashion designers picked up the idea and incorporated stars and stripes into their clothing designs, and soon those same young men and women who were arrested could look like patriotic super-heroes and -heroines. The analysis: If you can't lick 'em, make 'em fashionable!

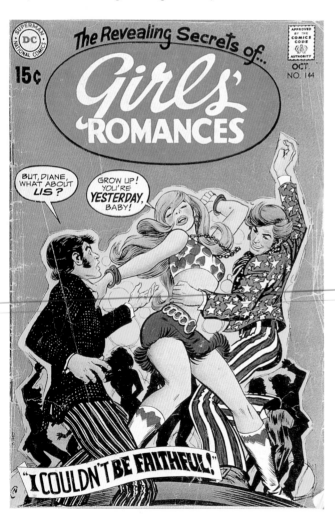

The cover of *Girls' Romances*, October, 1969, shows a pop-art couple; he in a flag outfit, she in God knows what!

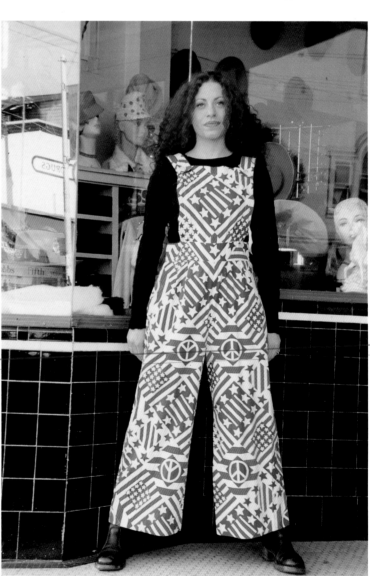

Flag designs and peace signs together on these cotton bellbottom overalls. No label. Courtesy Martini Mercantile.

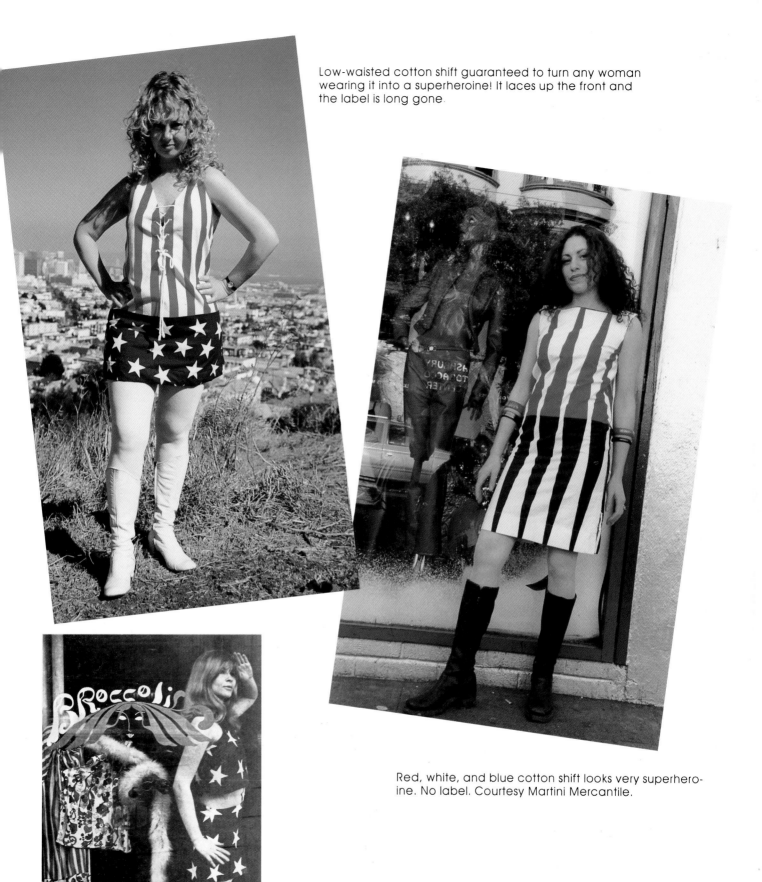

Low-waisted cotton shift guaranteed to turn any woman wearing it into a superheroine! It laces up the front and the label is long gone.

Red, white, and blue cotton shift looks very superheroine. No label. Courtesy Martini Mercantile.

The author, Trina Robbins, poses in the window of her East Village boutique, *Broccoli*, in 1968, wearing a dress she made from flag fabric.

Chapter Seven

Bellbottoms

Before about 1965, pants styles were straight, narrow, and ankle-high — they were the "floods" that the Beatles wore with their collarless jackets and Beatle boots. Then pants widened, at first staying narrow to at least the knees before widening out. Ultimately "bellbottoms" evolved to the extreme, widened from the hips, eventually becoming the very wide "elephant bells" of the early '70s. Although they sometimes had high-rise waistbands — a very attractive look — most of them were low-waisted "hip huggers." They looked best in bright, psychedelic patterns, and the pants hems were worn long, often dragging on the ground, which made for some pretty grungy bellbottoms' bottoms.

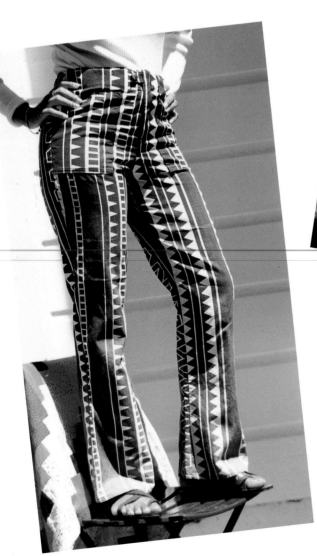

Bellbottoms decorated with black psychedelic swirls on white cotton. No label.

Really well made, fully-lined blue and white print cotton bellbottoms. The label says, "Swing West ski-wear by Raven, Sioux Falls, S.D.", but these don't look like ski-wear to me.

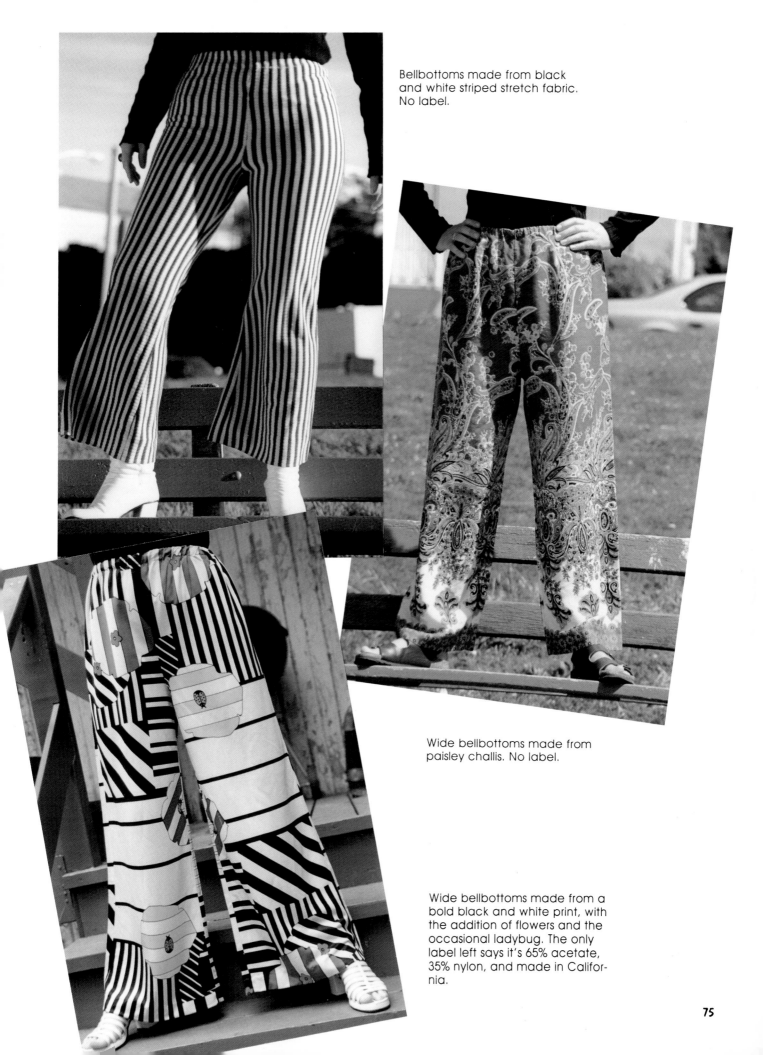

Bellbottoms made from black and white striped stretch fabric. No label.

Wide bellbottoms made from paisley challis. No label.

Wide bellbottoms made from a bold black and white print, with the addition of flowers and the occasional ladybug. The only label left says it's 65% acetate, 35% nylon, and made in California.

Beautiful high-waisted paisley-printed bellbottoms made from polyester chavacette. Label says, "Rowen."

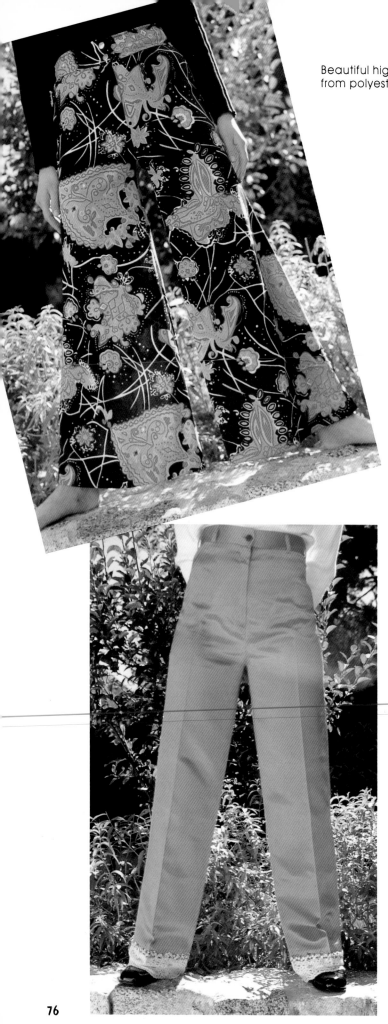

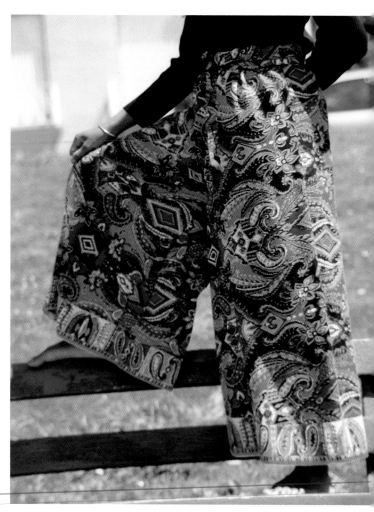

Super-wide "elephant bells", made from paisley challis with a paisley border sewn on at the hem, and with a self-belt, but no label.

These wonderful wide-legged lavender satin jeans come from the disco days of the 1970s, and have a wide band of gorgeous ecru lace at the cuff. The label says, "Los Angeles, California, J.J. & CO.", and tells us the pants are made from 100% acetate.

The Jumpsuit

The June 30, 1964 issue of *Look* magazine reported jumpsuits as the newest fashion and called them "the poolside pajama." "Fashion," they wrote, "is playing the pajama game....Seductive Sixties pajamas may remind a nostalgic few...of the theatrical Thirties."

Jumpsuits can be glamorous and fabulously flattering for the right figures.

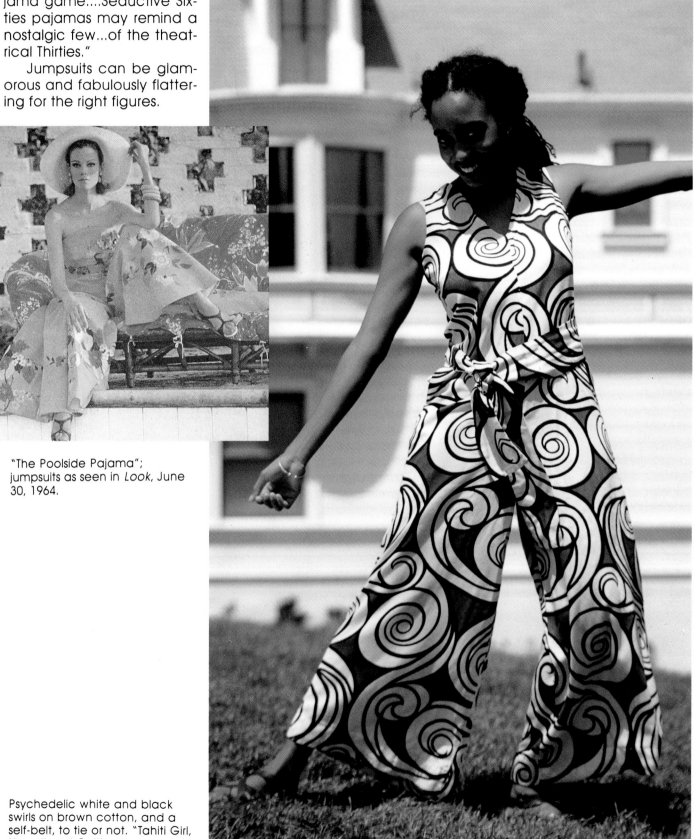

"The Poolside Pajama"; jumpsuits as seen in *Look*, June 30, 1964.

Psychedelic white and black swirls on brown cotton, and a self-belt, to tie or not. "Tahiti Girl, Hawaii and California."

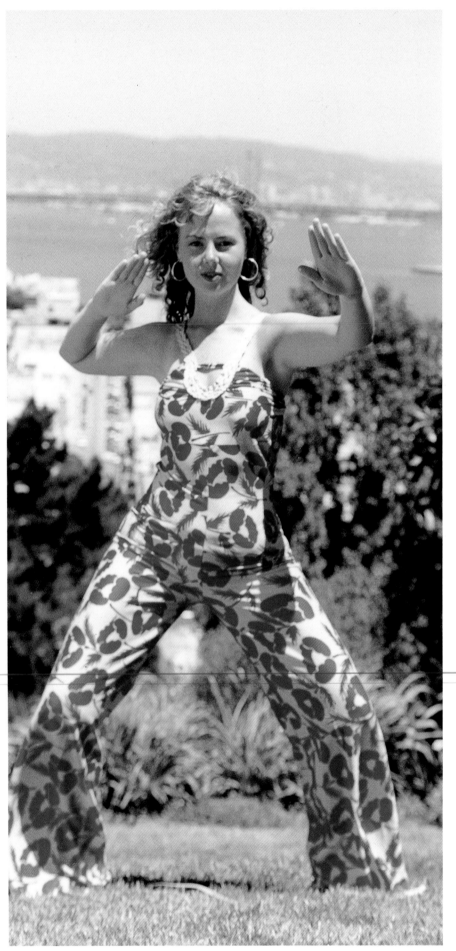

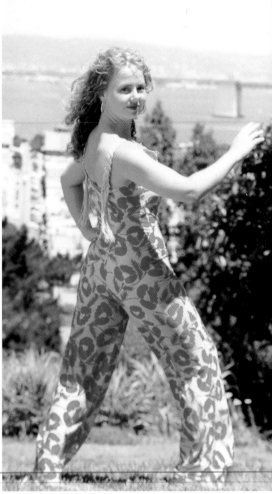

Two views of a 100% polyester jumpsuit beautifully trimmed with jute macramé shoulder straps. In back, the macramé straps hang down in fringe. "Estivo."

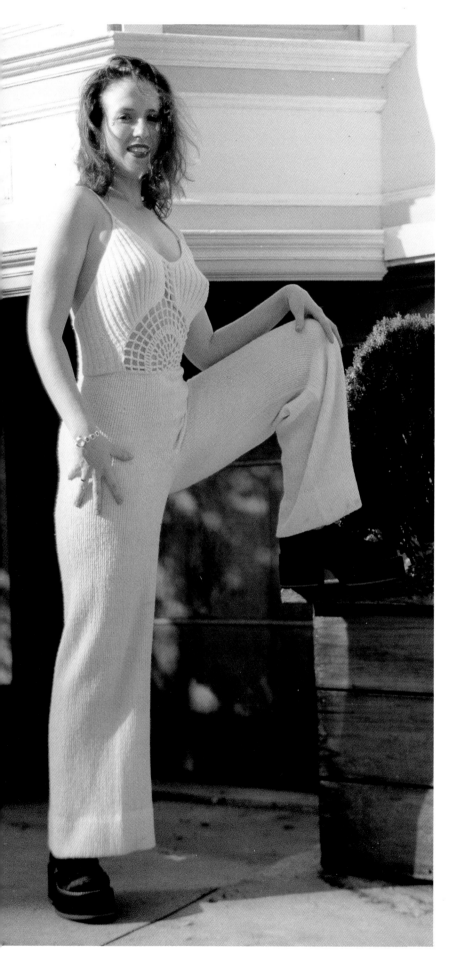

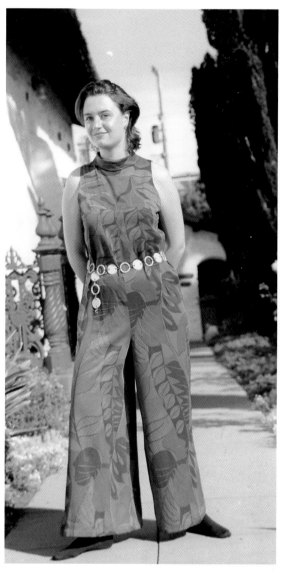

Lavender and dark blue leaves
on turquoise. No label.

Fabulous creme knit jumpsuit
with open midriff decorated
with crochet in a spiderweb
pattern. No label.

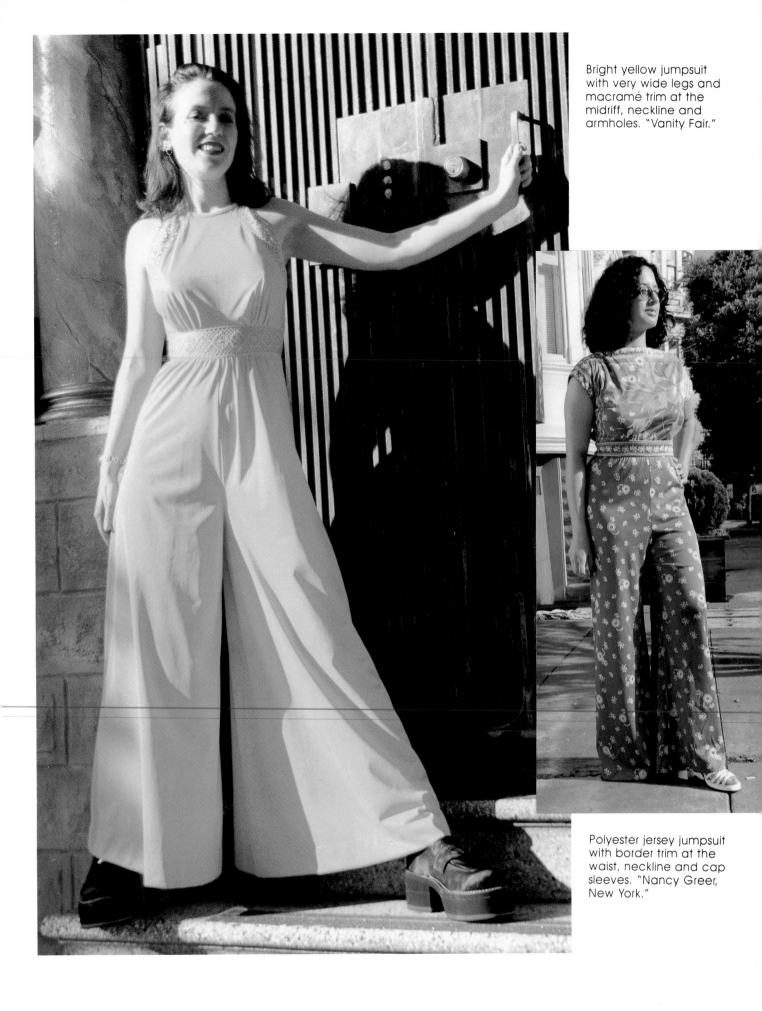

Bright yellow jumpsuit with very wide legs and macramé trim at the midriff, neckline and armholes. "Vanity Fair."

Polyester jersey jumpsuit with border trim at the waist, neckline and cap sleeves. "Nancy Greer, New York."

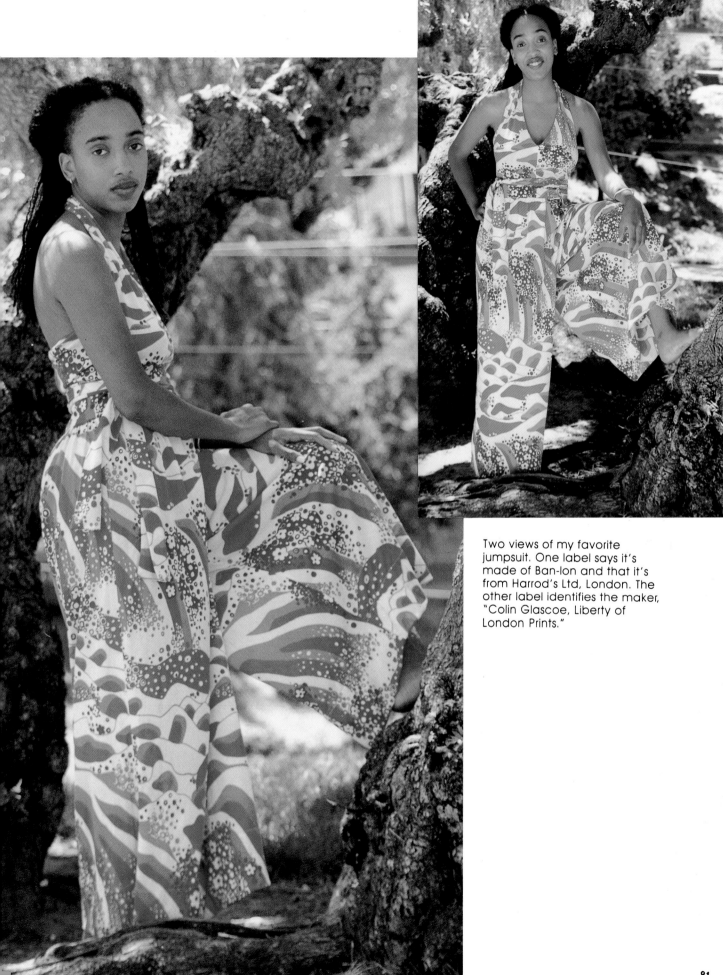

Two views of my favorite jumpsuit. One label says it's made of Ban-lon and that it's from Harrod's Ltd, London. The other label identifies the maker, "Colin Glascoe, Liberty of London Prints."

Chapter Eight

*F*abulous Flops

Some styles, like the paper dress, were an interesting idea from the paper companies looking for new markets, but they were just too silly to last. In the case of Rudy Gernreich's famous topless bathing suit, there wasn't much point trying to wear it to the beach where you'd only get arrested. Few women actually tried. Some styles were so unusual that once you had one, you didn't need another, and soon they went off the market! Those rarities are the real collectibles today; whether you can bring yourself to wear them is another question.

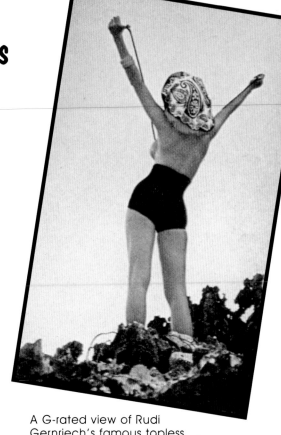

A G-rated view of Rudi Gernriech's famous topless bathing suit, from *look*, June 2, 1964.

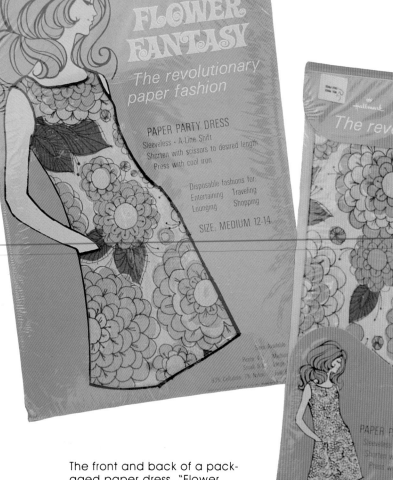

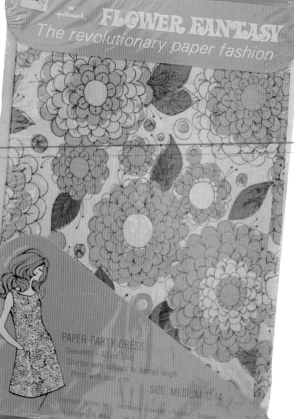

The front and back of a packaged paper dress. "Flower Fantasy" by Hallmark.

Hotpants

The name "hotpants" was coined by *Women's Wear Daily* in 1970, and the abbreviated hip-hugger shorts were popular for about a year. Worn with platform boots, they quickly became the uniform of some street prostitutes. Since most American women didn't really want to look like that, hotpants died young.

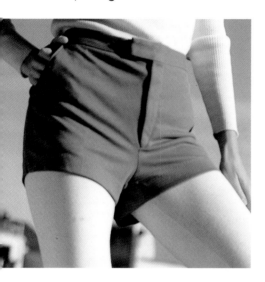

Poison green polyester double knit hotpants! The label says, "Your Advantage."

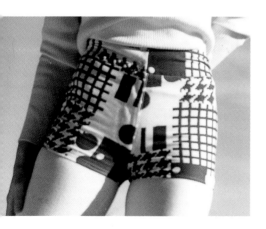

Very short cotton hotpants in a brown and white patchwork print. "Covella Sportswear."

Very cute polyester jersey hotpants playsuit. It's printed with little red and white sailboats and it zips up the front. No label.

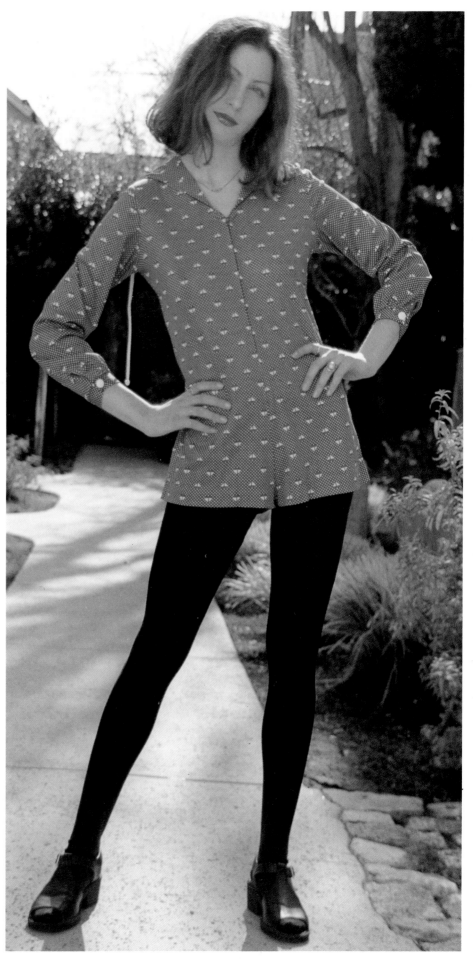

The Swirl Skirt

The graceful swirl skirt came to America from Europe around 1972 and took the country by storm. Cut in a unique pattern from a series of identical swirls, each of different fabrics, the swirl skirt was unusual and flattering. All anybody needed in their wardrobe was one, and once everybody had one, you couldn't give them away.

A spectacular swirl skirt whose panels are composed of four different prints. We paired it with this aqua crepe jacket with white pindots and white collar and cuffs, and a big red strawberry appliquéd on the collar. The jacket probably originally came with matching wide-legged pants, but it goes nicely with the skirt.

Swirl skirt made from two different plaids. The only part of the label left says it's made from 65% cotton, 35% acetate, and that it's made in California.

A contemporary swirl skirt made by me in 1995, from an old Butterick pattern.

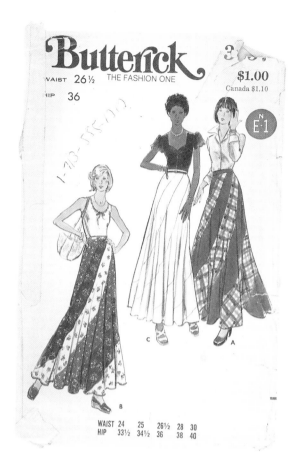

Butterick pattern for a swirl skirt. There's no date on the pattern, but it's probably from the early 1970s.

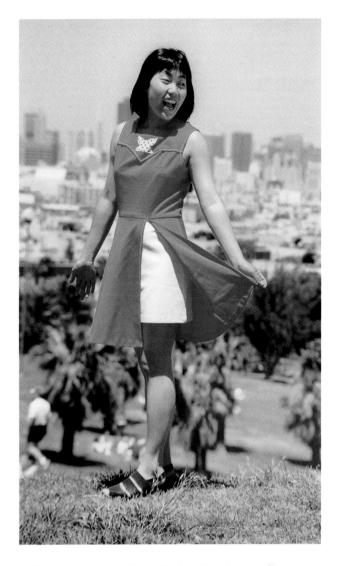

Red scooter dress with white topstitching, white shorts and red and white polkadotted butterfly appliquéd on the yoke. No label.

The Scooter Skirt

Also known as the "skort," the scooter skirt was one solution for what to wear under very short skirts — matching, attached shorts. The scooter skirt always featured slits to show off the shorts beneath, and the effect was leggy, perky and cute. Unfortunately, "skort" dresses posed a real problem for women in the ladies' room, especially if the temperature was cold. Need I say more?

Scooter skirt made from yellow and gray plaid polyester knit, with matching yellow shorts. "Sweet Swingers."

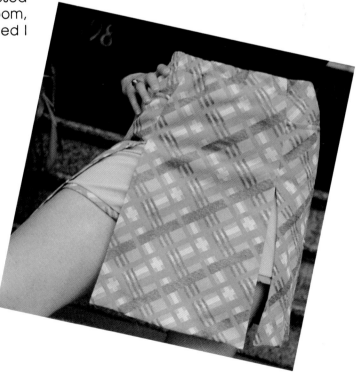

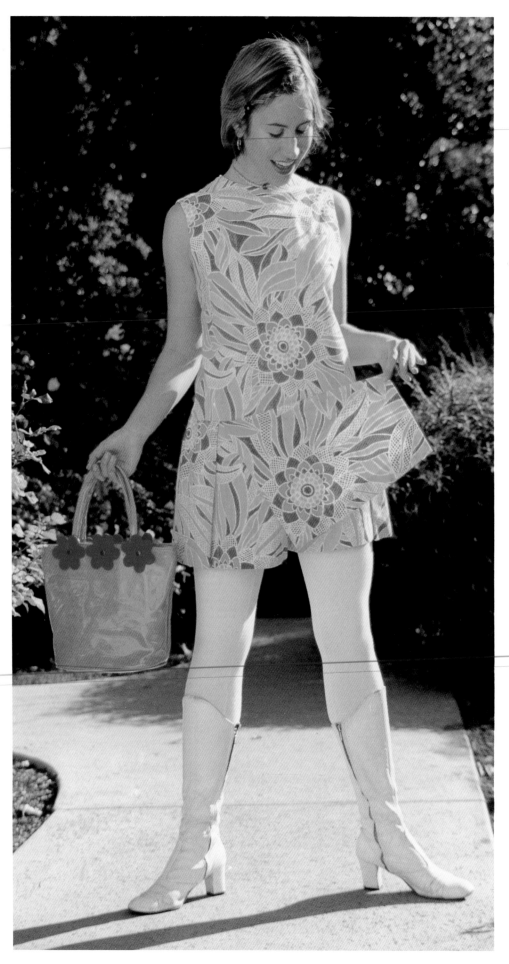

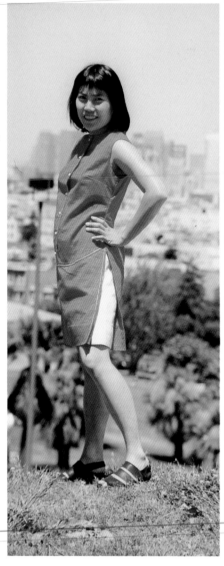

Another red scooter dress with white topstitching and white shorts! This one has a low waist and buttons down the front. "Junior West, California."

Very sunny yellow and orange scooter dress. No label.

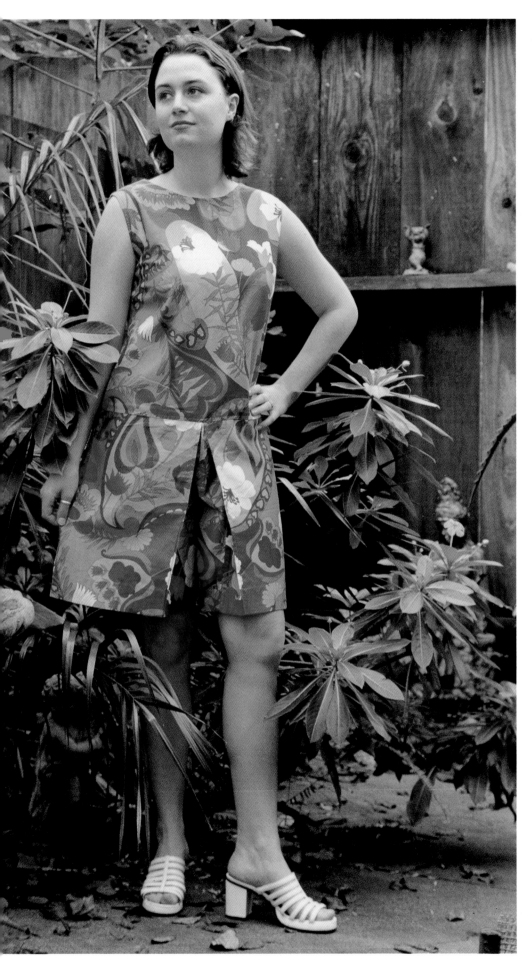

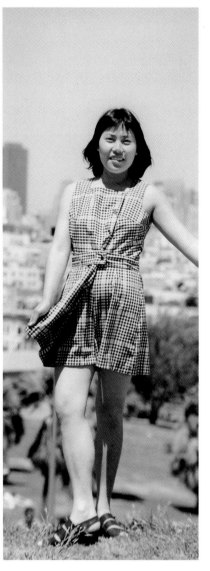

Black, white, and yellow plaid cotton scooter dress. No label.

Cotton scooter dress in a bright orange and green paisley print. "Alice Polynesian fashions."

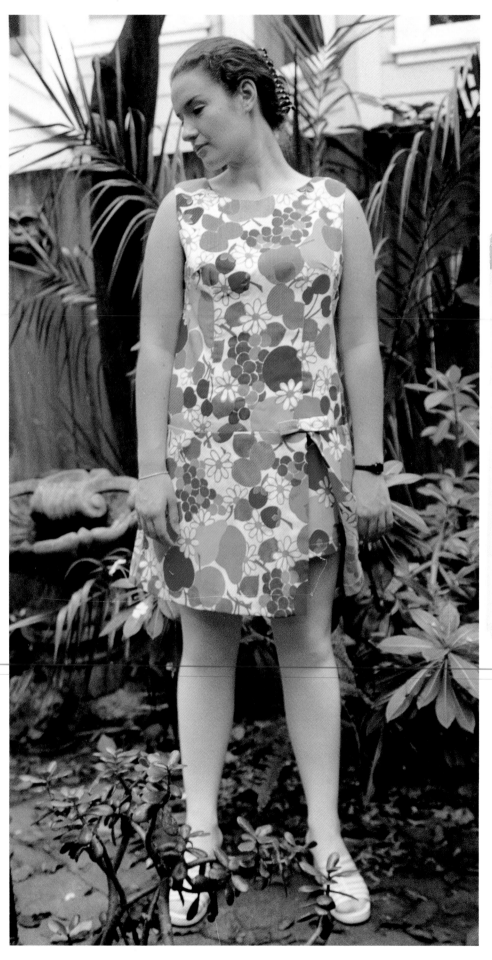

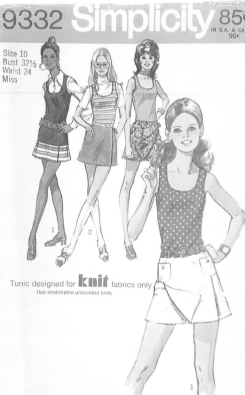

Simplicity pattern for a scooter skirt, dated 1971.

Very bright multi-colored flowers on white cotton scooter dress. No label.

Chapter Nine

Retro

The April, 1971 issue of *McCall's* magazine reported, "in 1971 nostalgia became a growth industry, with antique cars and antique movies, do-you-remember TV shows, trivia book clubs, and the like doing handsomely." But as early as the mid '60s, fashionable young women were already, like Suzanne in the Simon and Garfunkle song, "wearing rags and feathers from Salvation Army counters," not because they couldn't afford new clothes, but because they liked the look of the old ones. Savvy women dressed in '20s flapper dresses (which were much more available then) and shoulder-padded draped shapes of the '40s.

The popularity of the 1966 film *Bonnie and Clyde*, with authentic 1930s costuming, turned a growing interest in the style of the '20s and '30s into a national obsession. Toward the end of the '60s, the first vintage clothing shops started to spring up in major cities and soon the term Art Deco was on everybody's lips (although some of those people thought they were talking about a guy named Art!).

It didn't take long for the world of fashion to come up with brand new garments that looked as though they were thirty or forty years old, and these are known as "retro" designs. They featured high waistlines (like those of the 1930s), puffed sleeves, darker colors, white or cream-colored satin collars and cuffs, pin dots and pin stripes, and prints reminiscent of flapper cartoonist John Held, Junior. Some dresses were wrap-around styled, and many were knee length, like dresses from the '40s.

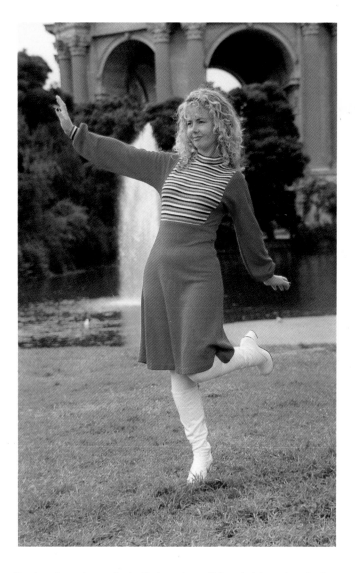

Rust colored acrylic knit dress has ribbed stripes inset at the top and at the cuffs. The label is mostly unreadable, but I suspect the dress is British, because I can read the words, "Height 158 cm."

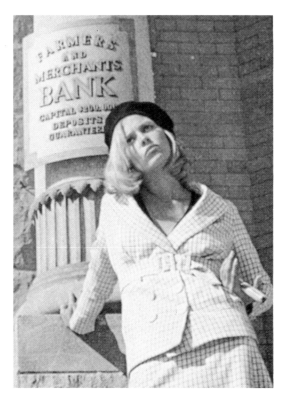

Faye Dunaway as Bonnie Parker in *Bonnie and Clyde*.

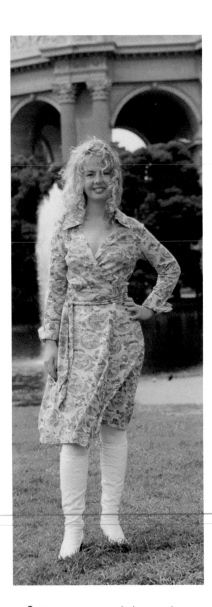

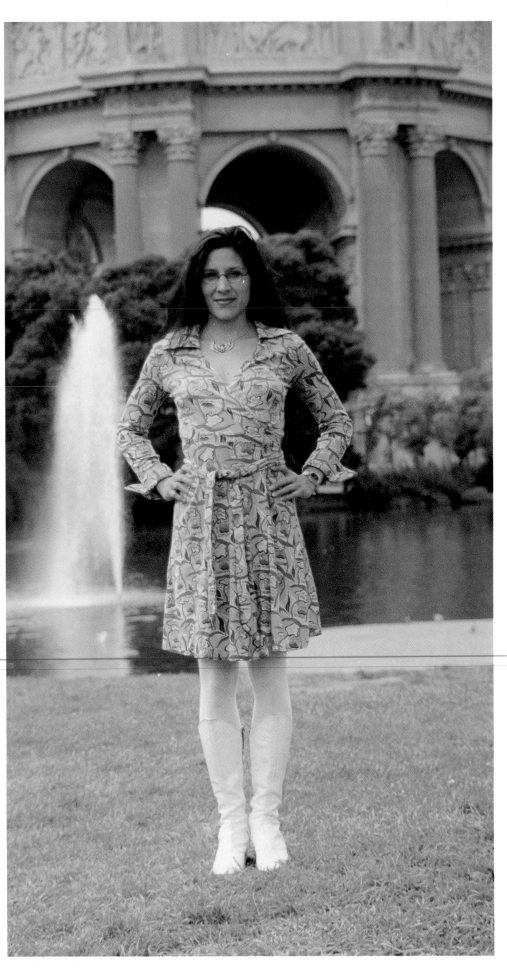

Two wraparound dresses by "Huk-A-Poo", both made from 100% acrylic jersey, both in exactly the same style, but different prints.

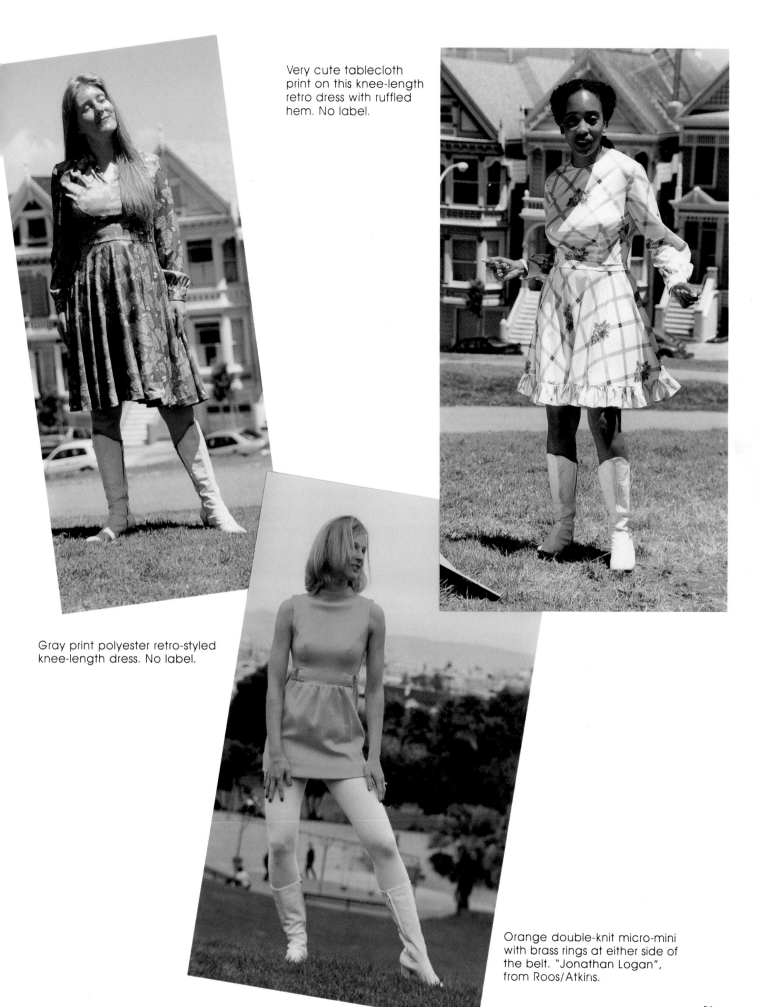

Very cute tablecloth print on this knee-length retro dress with ruffled hem. No label.

Gray print polyester retro-styled knee-length dress. No label.

Orange double-knit micro-mini with brass rings at either side of the belt. "Jonathan Logan", from Roos/Atkins.

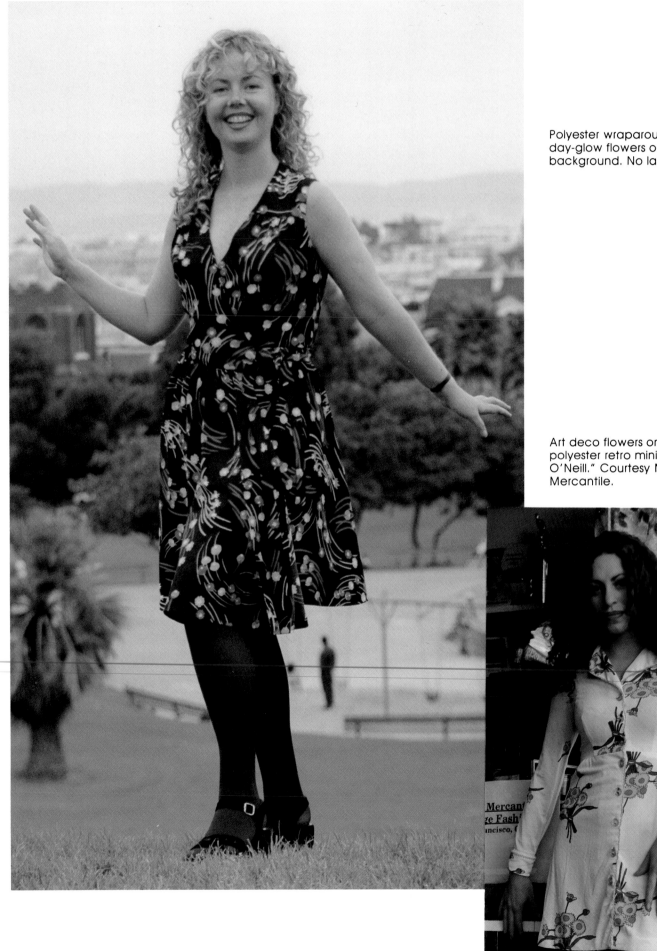

Polyester wraparound dress has day-glow flowers on a black background. No label.

Art deco flowers on a white polyester retro mini. "Patty O'Neill." Courtesy Martini Mercantile.

A band of white lace defines
the high waist on this retro mini
made from red houndstooth
print polyester jersey.

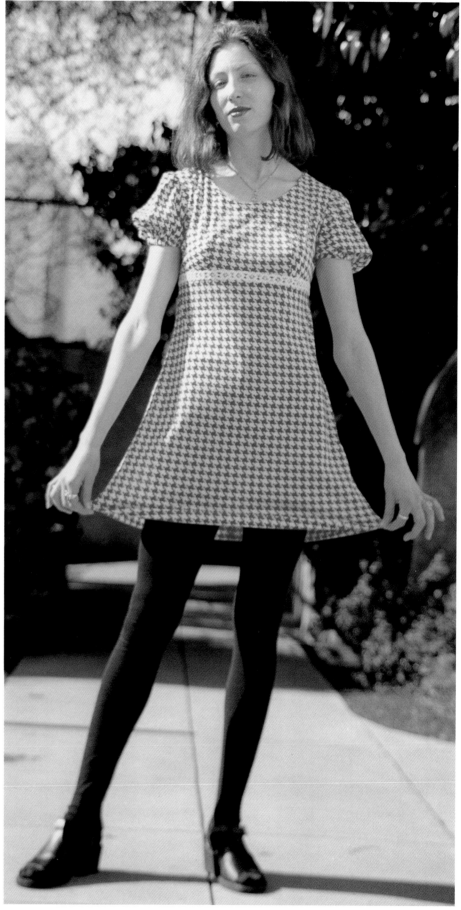

Dark green polyester retro mini
with contrasting collar and cuffs.
Courtesy Martini Mercantile.

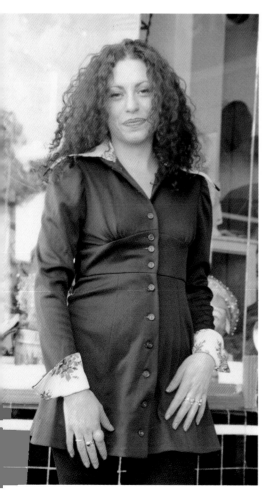

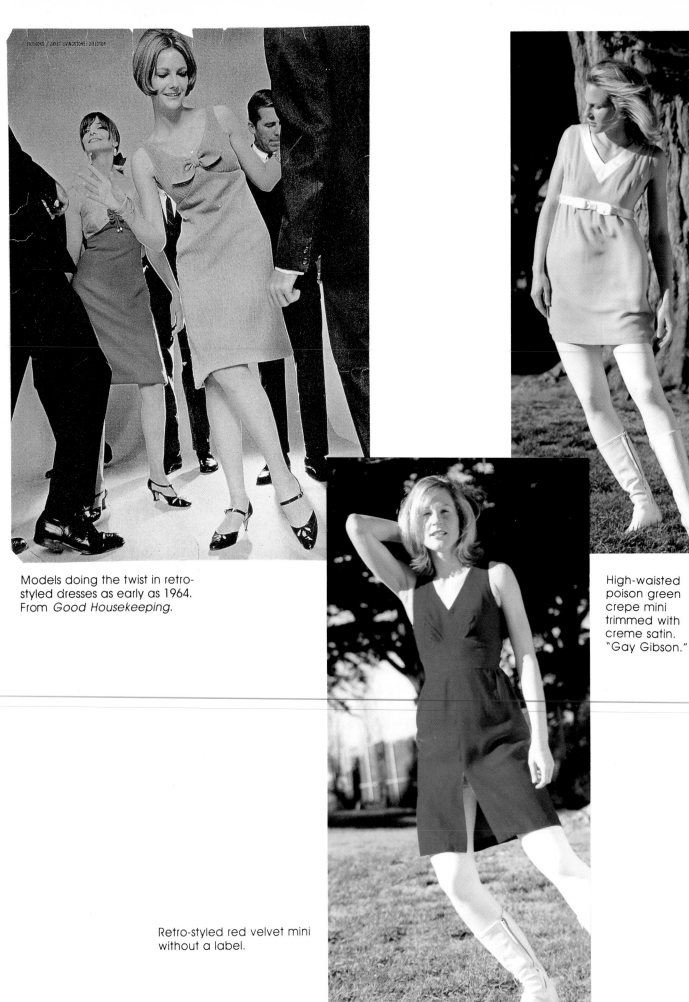

Models doing the twist in retro-styled dresses as early as 1964. From *Good Housekeeping*.

High-waisted poison green crepe mini trimmed with creme satin. "Gay Gibson."

Retro-styled red velvet mini without a label.

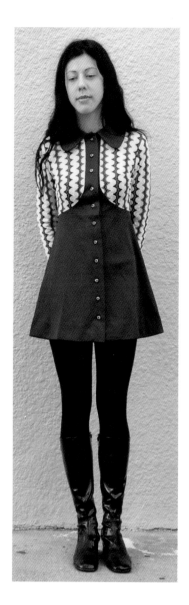

Polyester micro-mini has red, white, and blue stretch lace at bodice and sleeves, and little gold buttons down the front. "Staccato."

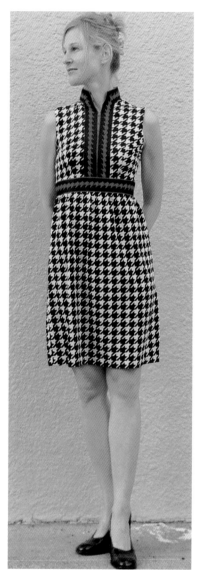

High-waisted polyester jersey dress in a dark green houndstooth print. No label.

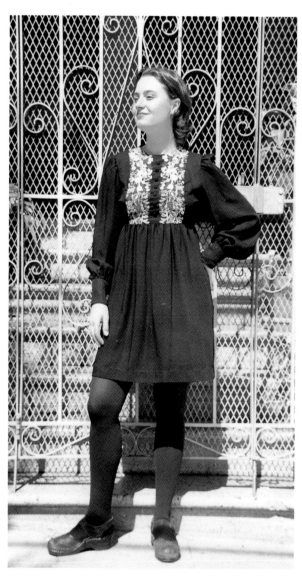

A high-waisted black crepe dress that will never go out of style. It has a row of self-covered buttons running down the bodice, between rows of embroidered flowers. The very full sleeves end in tight cuffs. No label.

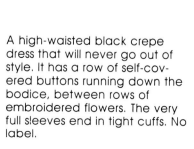

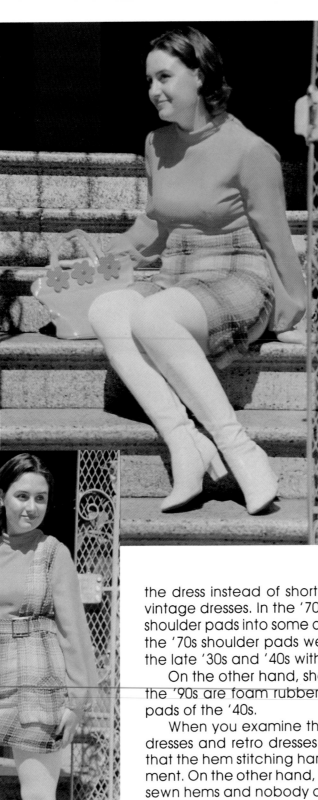

The blouse is bright orange crepe and the high-waisted plaid skirt is a synthetic wool imitation, but it's really a dress. Here it is with and without the matching long, belted vest.

Vintage vs. Retro

It is important to clarify the difference between "vintage" and "retro," a distinction I thought everyone already knew until the owner of a very good vintage clothing shop asked me the difference. **Original old garments are vintage. A new garment is retro** when it is made in the style of a vintage garment. Today, and throughout the 1990s, designers are making brand new clothing in the style of retro clothing from the '70s, which was in the style of clothing from the '30s! This is what I call "neo-retro."

Vintage clothing from the '40s and earlier will not be made from polyester fabric which was developed in the 1950s and widely available only in the '60s. In vintage clothing you will find silks, cottons, linens and wools, and a lot of rayon. Dresses with zippers have short zippers in a side seam at the waist area.

Retro dresses from the '70s were also often made from rayon, but they feature long zippers running down the back of the dress instead of short zippers at the waist as are found in vintage dresses. In the '70s, too, retro designers started putting shoulder pads into some of their clothing for a vintage look, but the '70s shoulder pads were much smaller than the ones from the late '30s and '40s with white stuffing.

On the other hand, shoulder pads in neo-retro dresses from the '90s are foam rubber and even bigger than the shoulder pads of the '40s.

When you examine the hems, you'll find that both vintage dresses and retro dresses from the '70s have wide hems, and that the hem stitching hardly shows on the right side of the garment. On the other hand, neo-retro dresses have tiny, machine-sewn hems and nobody cares anymore if the stitches show. Be careful, though, not to judge the age of a garment solely by its hem, because many hems have been taken up or let down.

Speaking of hems, this is a good opportunity to condemn the unfortunate practice of cutting long dresses into minis. Far too many potentially beautiful dresses from the '30s were ruined beyond repair when hippie women cut them into minis in the '60s, and now I see people doing the same thing to long dresses from the '60s and '70s. Please! These dresses were designed to be long, and cutting them spoils the original lines. If you spy a great granny in a thrift shop, but really wanted a mini, fight the urge to cut it, and leave it for someone who will appreciate it in its original length. Of course, hems are another story. If your long dress is dragging on the ground, you're stepping on your bellbottoms, or your mini reaches below your knees, by all means hem them. As a short person, I find it necessary to hem all my vintage finds, and my new ones, too.

Finally, when in doubt about the age of a garment, check the labels. If they still exist in the garment, labels on pre-'60s clothing tend to be pretty straightforward, such as "A Dorothy Original, made in Oz." By the mid-'60s, many labels brightened up with "rock and roll-style" lettering and perhaps even "hip" embroidered art, and the wording might be more flip: "Dotty Casuals, from Sunny Oz." Names on '90s labels almost sound like rock groups, like "Stars Over Oz." Unless they're made in Paris or elsewhere abroad, most vintage clothing will have union labels that say "Made in America."

Waistlines

Retro dresses of the early 1960s were just variations on the shift; they hearkened back to the flapper days of the '20s and featured low waistlines. In 1964, *Good Housekeeping* magazine featured a spread showing models doing what appears to be the twist, in empire-waisted slip dresses that reflect the '30s. By the end of the '60s, the high-waisted look of the 30s had come to stay through much of the '70s.

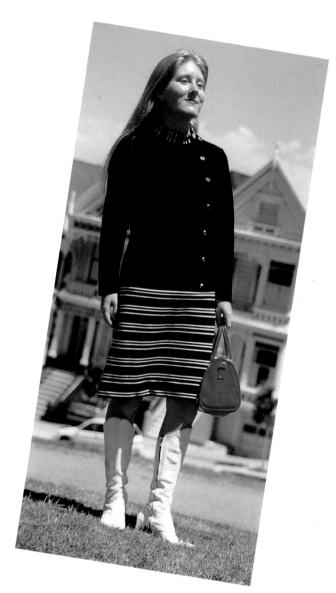

Low-waisted black and white double-knit dress has brass buttons down the side. "Bleeker Street."

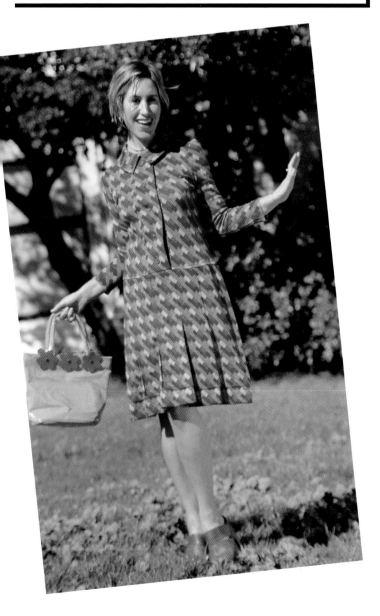

This low-waisted dress with a pleated skirt hearkens back to the 1920s, with its woven wine and gold Art Deco pattern. The label says, "Courtelle" and tells us it came from Lord and Taylor, and was made in France from fabric that is 25% wool and 75% acrylic.

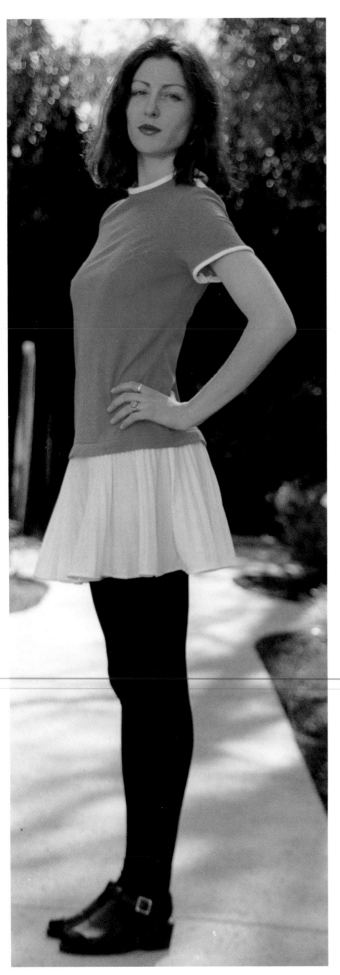

The bright orange top of this really cute low-waisted dress is banded in white at the neckline, sleeves, and at the shoulders, where it closes with little decorative zippers. The white skirt is permanently pleated.

Low-waisted dress has a white top, red band at the hip and blue permanently pleated skirt.

More flag colors on this knit dress with a striped permanently pleated skirt, and matching binding at the neckline. "Sacony Ciella."

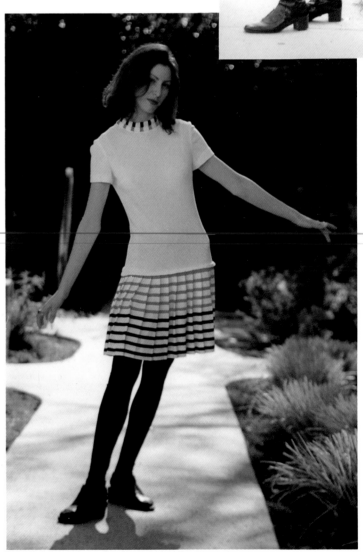

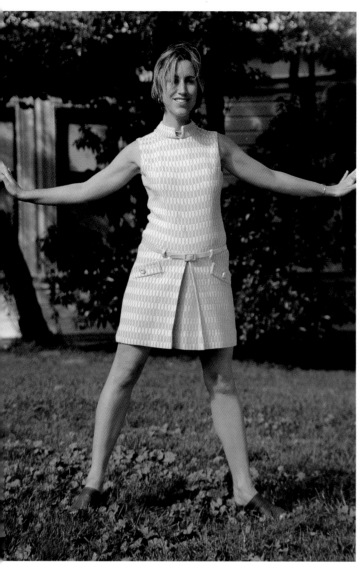

Low-waisted mini is made from loosely-woven yellow and white wool, belts at the hip with its own yellow belt, has buttoned pocket flaps and an inverted pleat in the skirt. No label.

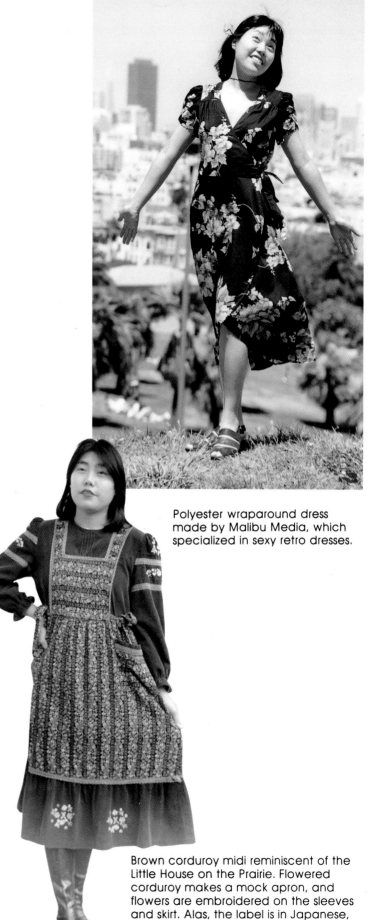

Polyester wraparound dress made by Malibu Media, which specialized in sexy retro dresses.

Midis and Maxis

The midi-skirt, which reached about mid-calf length, was a retro look inspired by clothing shown in the 1966 film *Doctor Zhivago*. Midis really came into their own towards the end of that decade and were widely worn in the early '70s; they looked great with high boots. The maxi-skirt's popularity originated in the late '60s and they went down to the ankles. The difference between a maxi dress and a granny dress is in their styling, with granny dresses being earlier versions of the maxis.

Brown corduroy midi reminiscent of the Little House on the Prairie. Flowered corduroy makes a mock apron, and flowers are embroidered on the sleeves and skirt. Alas, the label is in Japanese, so I don't know what it says!

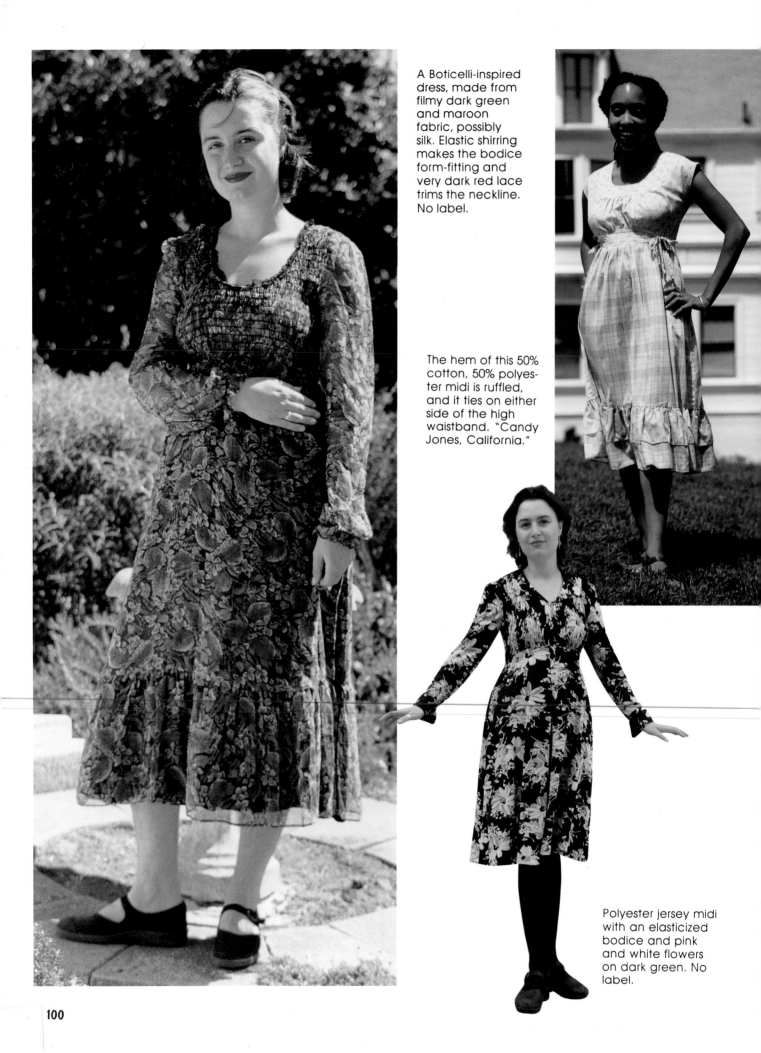

A Boticelli-inspired dress, made from filmy dark green and maroon fabric, possibly silk. Elastic shirring makes the bodice form-fitting and very dark red lace trims the neckline. No label.

The hem of this 50% cotton, 50% polyester midi is ruffled, and it ties on either side of the high waistband. "Candy Jones, California."

Polyester jersey midi with an elasticized bodice and pink and white flowers on dark green. No label.

Another maxi-dress that looks like two-pieces. The top is a solid black ribbed knit and the skirt is checkerboard- and flower print chavacette. Little buttons close the top. "Goldworm, made in Italy, 100% polyester."

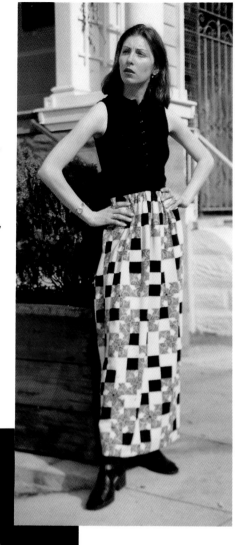

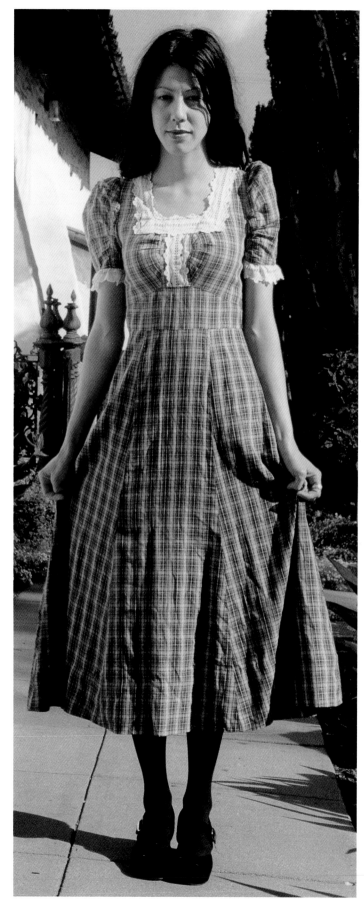

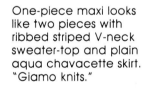

One-piece maxi looks like two pieces with ribbed striped V-neck sweater-top and plain aqua chavacette skirt. "Giamo knits."

One of my favorites, this retro dress really looks like it came from about 1938! I love the lace trim at the square neckline, bodice and cuffs of the poufed sleeves. "Foxy Lady, San Francisco."

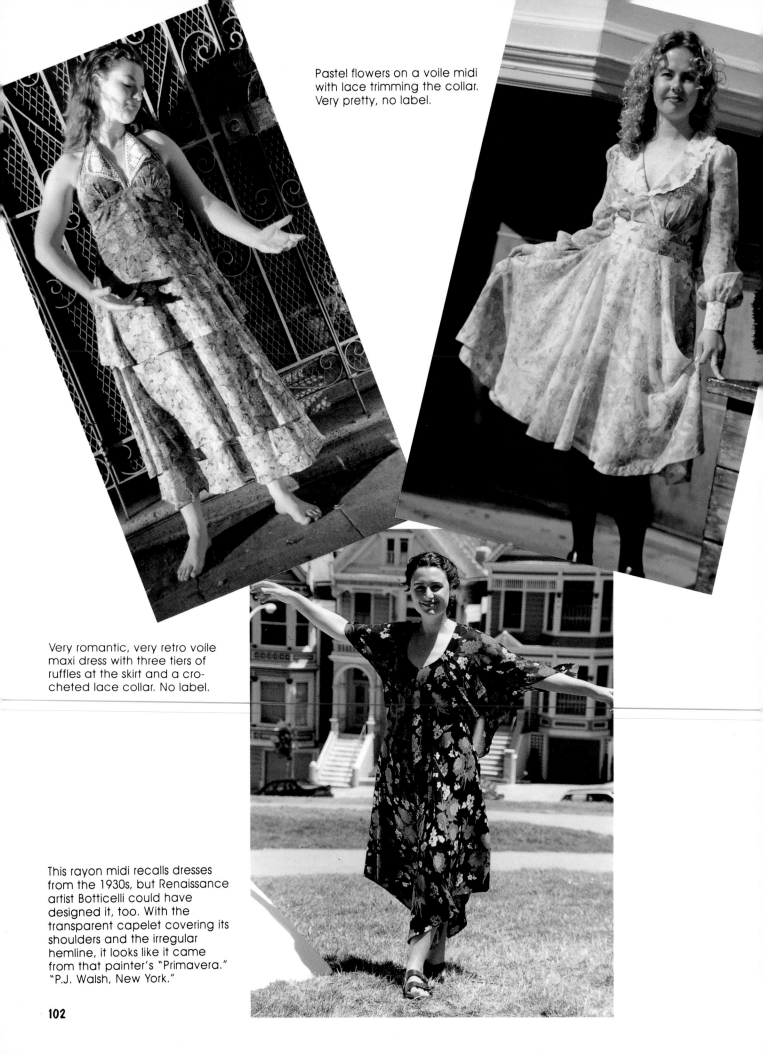

Pastel flowers on a voile midi with lace trimming the collar. Very pretty, no label.

Very romantic, very retro voile maxi dress with three tiers of ruffles at the skirt and a crocheted lace collar. No label.

This rayon midi recalls dresses from the 1930s, but Renaissance artist Botticelli could have designed it, too. With the transparent capelet covering its shoulders and the irregular hemline, it looks like it came from that painter's "Primavera." "P.J. Walsh, New York."

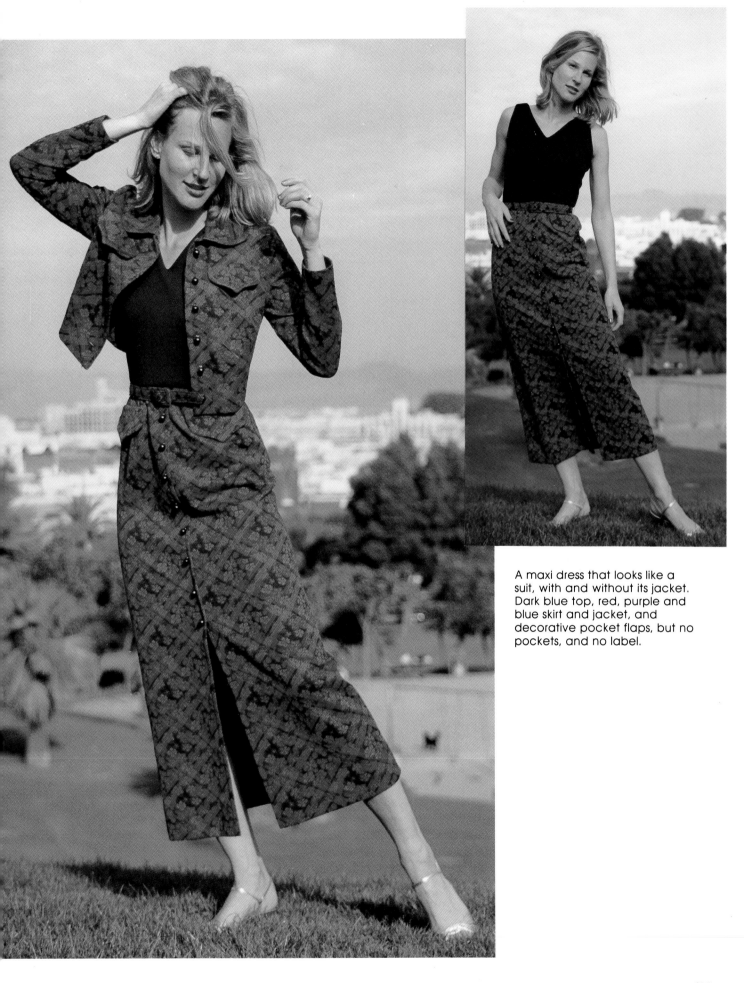

A maxi dress that looks like a suit, with and without its jacket. Dark blue top, red, purple and blue skirt and jacket, and decorative pocket flaps, but no pockets, and no label.

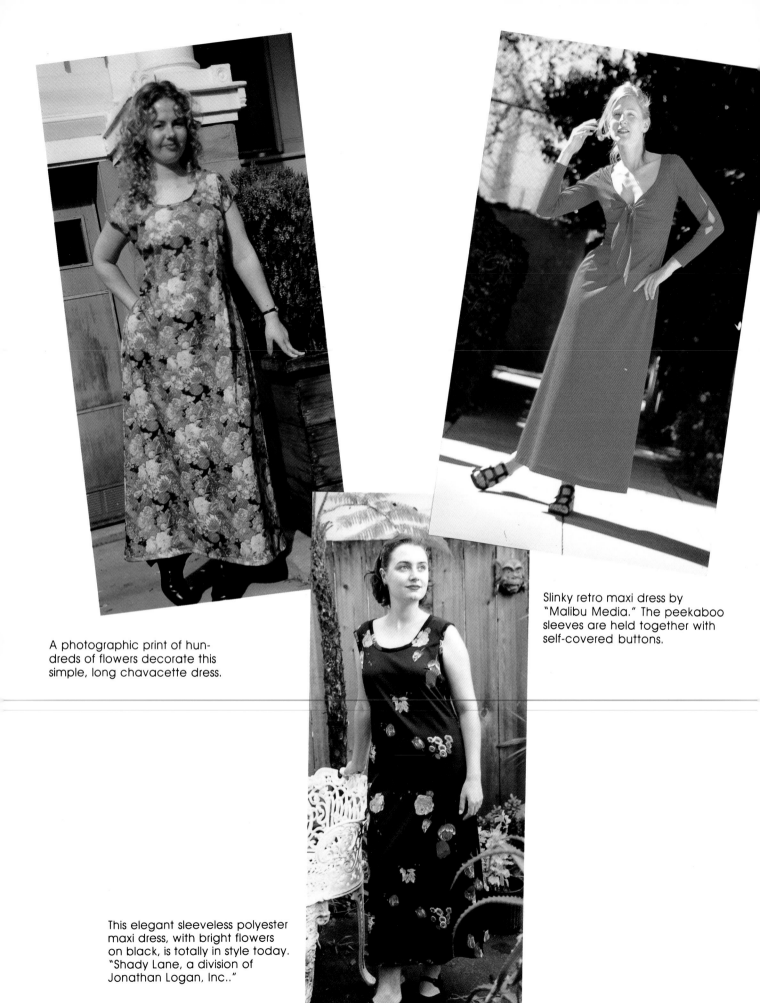

A photographic print of hundreds of flowers decorate this simple, long chavacette dress.

Slinky retro maxi dress by "Malibu Media." The peekaboo sleeves are held together with self-covered buttons.

This elegant sleeveless polyester maxi dress, with bright flowers on black, is totally in style today. "Shady Lane, a division of Jonathan Logan, Inc.."

The Jean Harlow Dress

One of the most popular, and sexiest, retro looks for sundresses and party dresses was inspired by the slinky, satin, halter-necked gowns worn by platinum bombshell film star Jean Harlow in her 1930s films. Retro versions of her dresses were made in any number of different fabrics besides satin, and they actually looked best in bright day-glow colors and psychedelic prints that glowed under a black light for disco dancing.

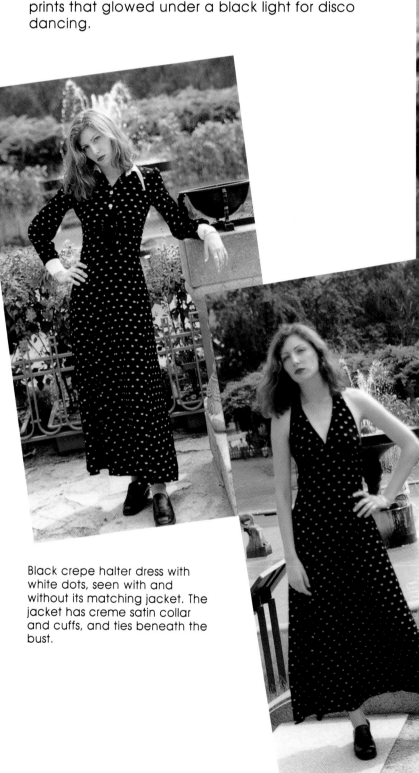

One of my favorites — a retro halter dress covered with extremely bright flowers in every color imaginable. No label.

Black crepe halter dress with white dots, seen with and without its matching jacket. The jacket has creme satin collar and cuffs, and ties beneath the bust.

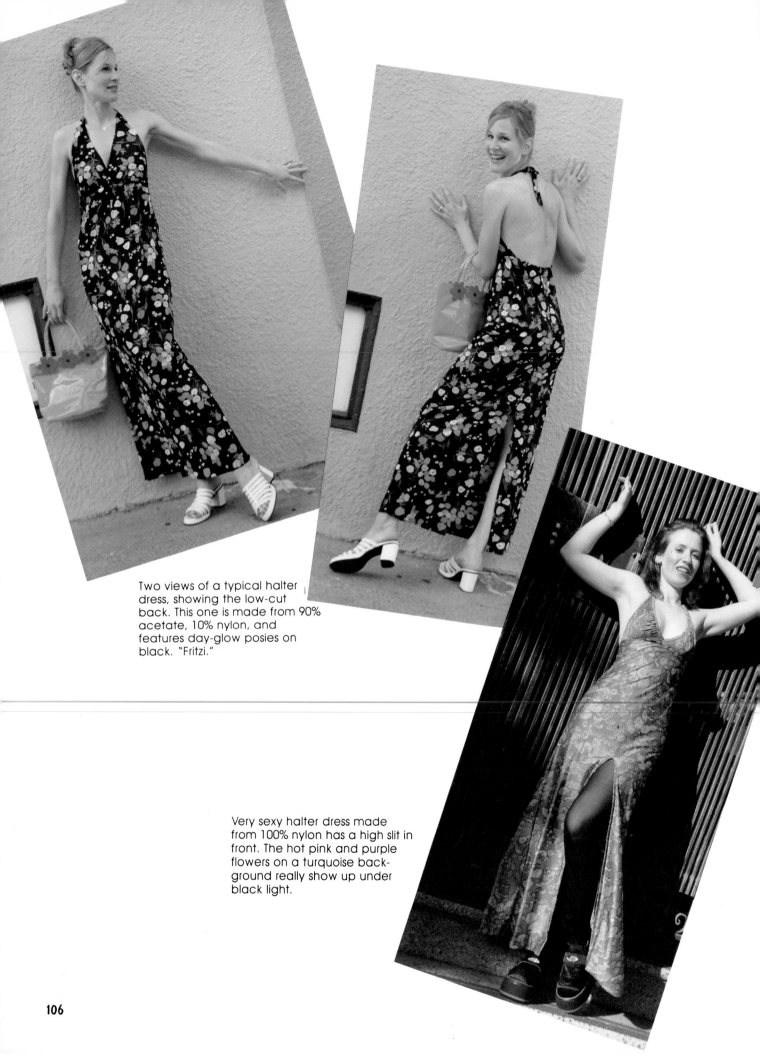

Two views of a typical halter dress, showing the low-cut back. This one is made from 90% acetate, 10% nylon, and features day-glow posies on black. "Fritzi."

Very sexy halter dress made from 100% nylon has a high slit in front. The hot pink and purple flowers on a turquoise background really show up under black light.

Chapter Ten
Hawaii

Some of the brightest, happiest, and most collectible fashions of the '60s and '70s were made in styles and from fabrics that were designed in Hawaii. From mini to maxi in length, these clothes were inspired by Hawaiian muumuus with added '60s and '70s styling. Long, graceful dresses called Holokus were among the prettiest. Some had raised waistlines, some had floating panels in the back, and some daring halter-top dresses had no back at all. Because they were resort fashions, Hawaiian style clothes were meant for vacation rather than for everyday wear and they got pretty fanciful. The resort clothing is grouped together here and some of the outfits were made in tropical California or Florida rather than Hawaii. This reflects the greater competition that evolved for the Hawaiian style market.

Although a good many Hawaiian styles were made from polyester, the typical fabric for Hawaiian resort clothing was a heavy textured cotton, cotton blend, or good imitation called bark cloth. The idea was for the fabric to resemble tapa, the original Hawaiian cloth, made from the bark of the mulberry tree. Whatever the fabric, it's always brightly printed — there are no solids in Hawaii! Sometimes the print resembles batik, sometimes the traditional Hawaiian style of white flowers on a bright background, and sometimes just wild, psychedelic flowers, but always bright. Unfortunately, there is a costume-like look to most of these fashions (they were, after all, costumes of a sort originally) that makes them hard to wear in a modern city. I either save my vintage Hawaiian clothes for trips to Hawaii or wear them in the evenings and for special occasions.

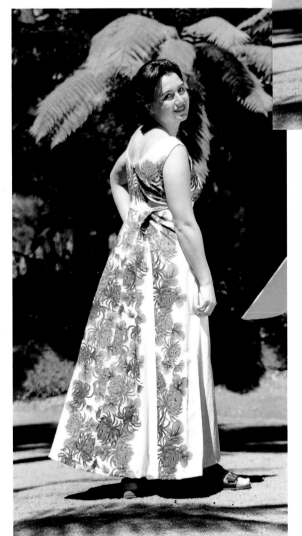

Two views of the long Hawaiian dress, showing the straight-cut front and the full back, almost a train. It's made from 100% cotton bark cloth, and the label says, "Ui-Makai, made in Hawaii."

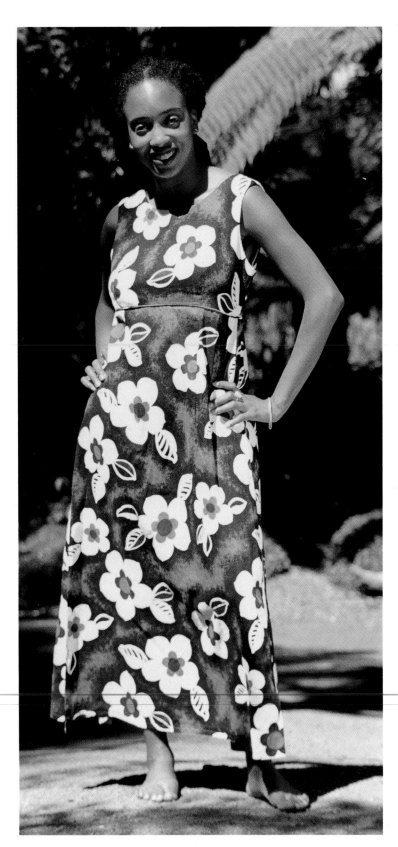

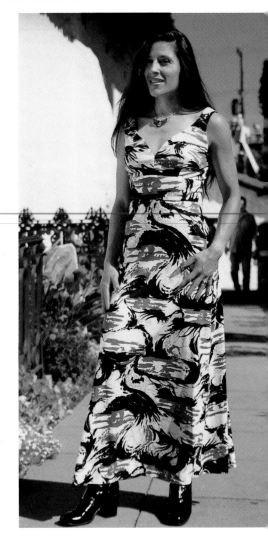

100% polyester, retro-styled Hawaiian dress has a psyche-delic flower design on dark green. No label.

Big white flowers on a bright blue background adorn this high-waisted dress of 100% cotton bark cloth. The label says only, "Made in Hawaii."

The abstract dark blue and green print of this long tropical-style polyester jersey dress looks like it might be waves. "Cirette of California."

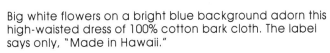

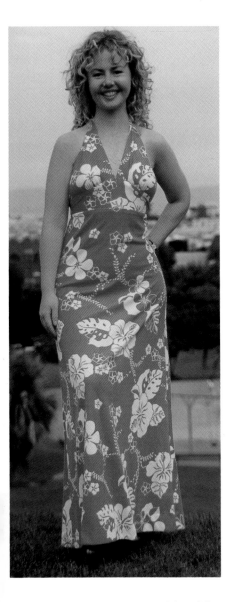

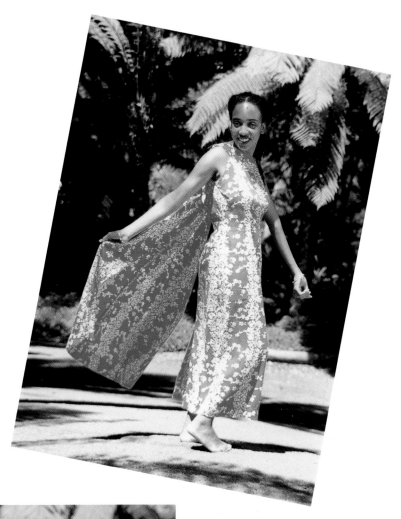

I love this dress with its big white flowers on bright orange, because it reminds me of old Dorothy Lamour movies! "Kiholo Fashions, made and styled in Hawaii."

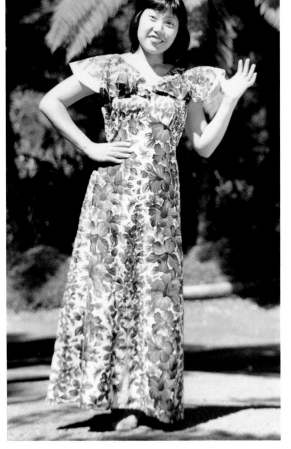

This long, fitted Hawaiian dress is made from 100% acetate, but it looks like cotton. It features white flowers on bright orange, with a floating panel in back. The cute label has a hula girl embroidered on it, and says, "fashioned by Hukilau Fashions, Honolulu."

This high-waisted dress with ruffled sleeves is reminiscent of the holokus of the 1930s. "Haleaka Fashions, made in Hawaii."

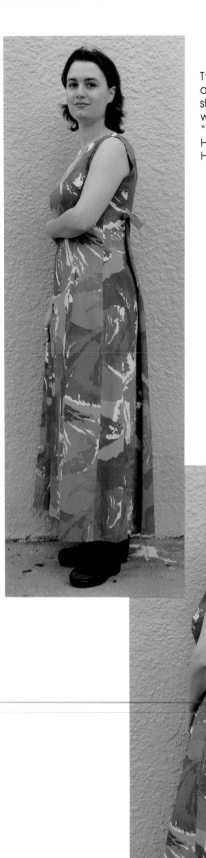

Two views of a 100% acrylic blue and green Hawaiian dress, showing the full back, trimmed with two little bows. It's a "Casual Aire", from Reef Towers, Hawaiian Village Outrigger Hotel, Honolulu.

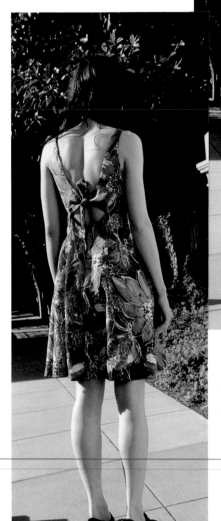

Two views of a cute blue and green sundress, showing how it ties at the open back. "Kimo's Polynesian Shop."

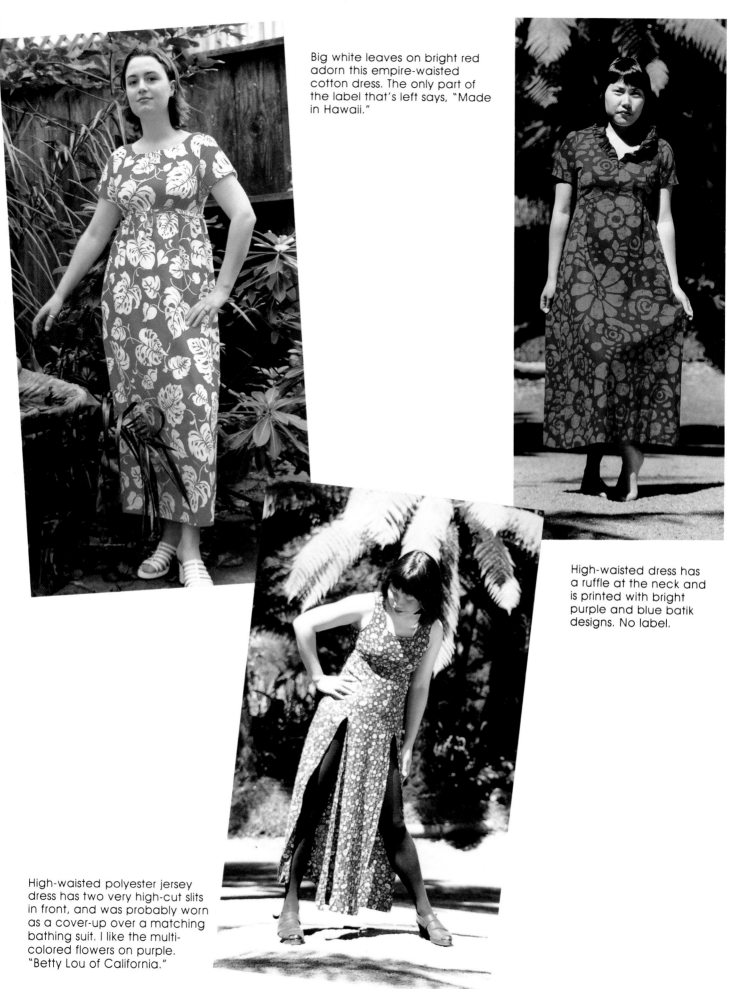

Big white leaves on bright red adorn this empire-waisted cotton dress. The only part of the label that's left says, "Made in Hawaii."

High-waisted dress has a ruffle at the neck and is printed with bright purple and blue batik designs. No label.

High-waisted polyester jersey dress has two very high-cut slits in front, and was probably worn as a cover-up over a matching bathing suit. I like the multi-colored flowers on purple. "Betty Lou of California."

111

Asian Styling

Chinese-inspired styling abounds in Hawaiian resort clothing, influenced by the large Asian population of those beautiful islands. You'll find lots of mandarin collars, frog closings, and wide kimono sleeves, all very flattering and graceful.

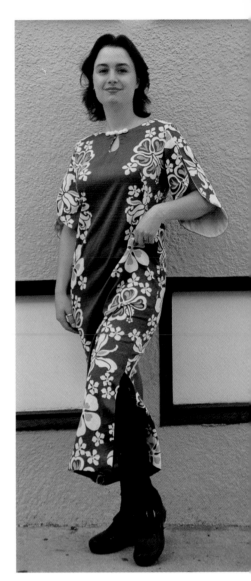

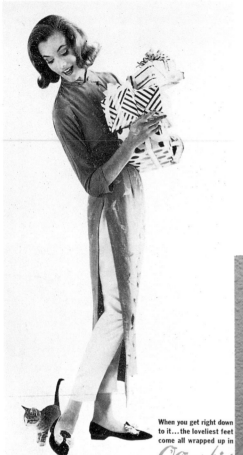

This high-slit, flowered Chinese dress was worn over straight-cut pants as leisure wear in the early 1960s. From *Glamour*, November, 1961.

When you get right down to it...the loveliest feet come all wrapped up in *OOmphies*

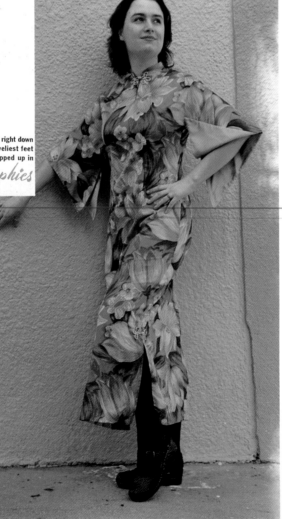

Big white flowers run down the sides of this dark green Chinese-inspired dress. The kimono sleeves are lined with white to match the frog closing at the keyhole neckline. "Sears Hawaiian Fashions."

This is my favorite Chinese-inspired Hawaiian dress! There are gold frogs at the side slits and the Mandarin collar. The kimono sleeves are lined in mint green, and I love the bright flower print. No label, who cares?

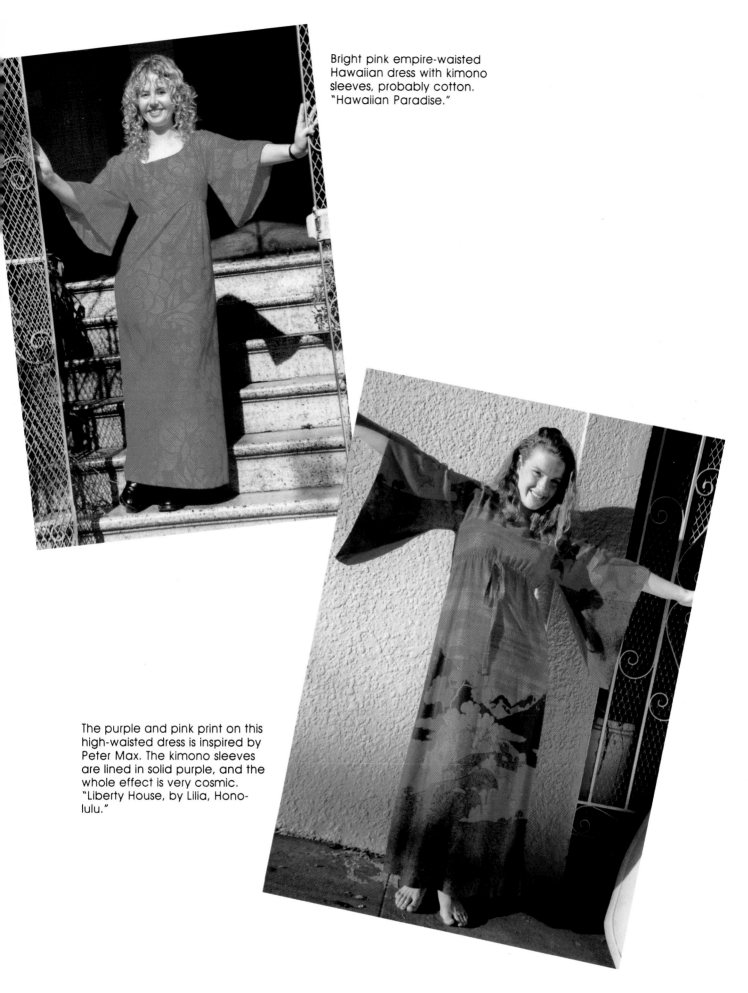

Bright pink empire-waisted Hawaiian dress with kimono sleeves, probably cotton. "Hawaiian Paradise."

The purple and pink print on this high-waisted dress is inspired by Peter Max. The kimono sleeves are lined in solid purple, and the whole effect is very cosmic. "Liberty House, by Lilia, Honolulu."

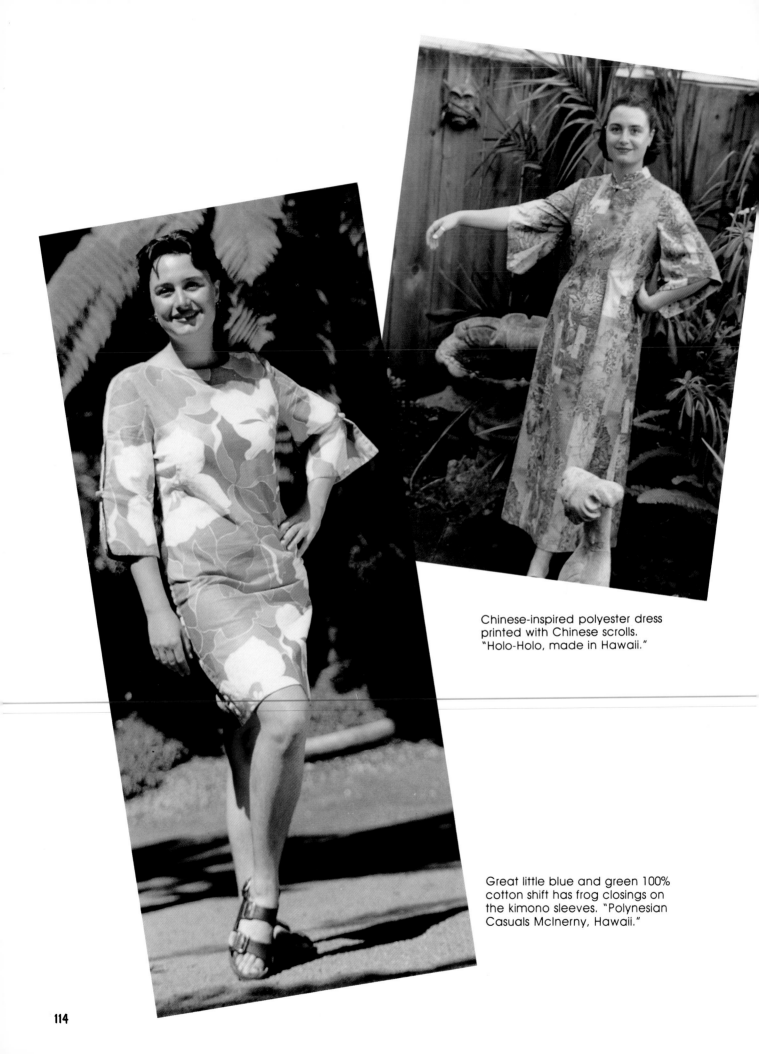

Chinese-inspired polyester dress printed with Chinese scrolls. "Holo-Holo, made in Hawaii."

Great little blue and green 100% cotton shift has frog closings on the kimono sleeves. "Polynesian Casuals McInerny, Hawaii."

Chapter Eleven
Denim

That old workhorse, cotton denim, which had previously been seen primarily on farmers in the form of overalls and on teenagers in the form of dungarees, got all duded up in the late '60s. As was true with patchwork, the reasons for denim's popularity in the '60s was partly political and partly philosophical. Denim was like folk music in that it talked about the common working man and simple, down-home life. Calico patchwork and lace were added to denim by fashion designer Jessica McClintock of Gunne sax and proved to be a marriage made in heaven. By the '70s, popular designers were adding glitter to denim in the forms of silver and gold piping to trim bellbottom jeans and studs to adorn denim jackets. Denim went disco!

Advertisement for a denim jumpsuit from *Seventeen*, October, 1976.

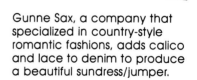

Gunne Sax, a company that specialized in country-style romantic fashions, adds calico and lace to denim to produce a beautiful sundress/jumper.

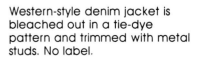

Western-style denim jacket is bleached out in a tie-dye pattern and trimmed with metal studs. No label.

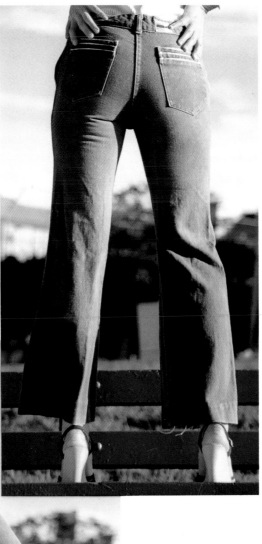

Two views of denim bellbottomed jeans trimmed with silver piping on the side and back pockets. "MGR."

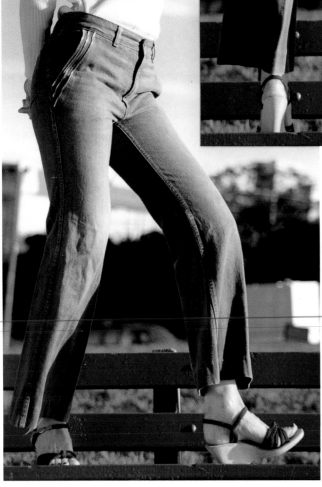

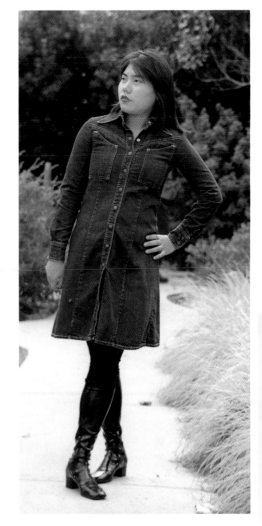

Around 1977, everybody had one of these denim coatdresses! This one fastens down the front with fancy brass snaps. No label.

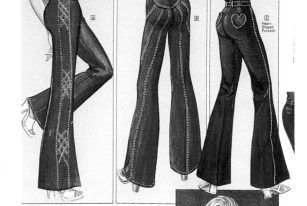

Fancy bellbottomed jeans from the 1978 *Frederick's of Hollywood* catalogue.

Chapter Twelve

Some Famous Designers

Clothing with the label of a famous designer from twenty-five or thirty years ago (or earlier!) is collectible today. I know a young woman who collects designer scarves which are easier to find and less expensive than designer dresses. A few of the popular fashion designers from the '60s and '70s are mentioned below:

Emilio Pucci

A designer who will always be associated with the '60s was Emilio Pucci, born the Marchese di Barsento in Naples, Italy, in 1914. A descendant of Russian nobility, he died in Florence in 1990. His brilliantly printed little jersey shifts were a favorite of the international jet set in the '60s, and were widely copied throughout the decade. He also designed affordable underwear, which today can easily be worn as outerwear. Vintage Pucci designs probably cost more than any other fashions from the same period, so collecting his lower-priced shortie nightgowns and slips, and wearing them as dresses, is a good idea.

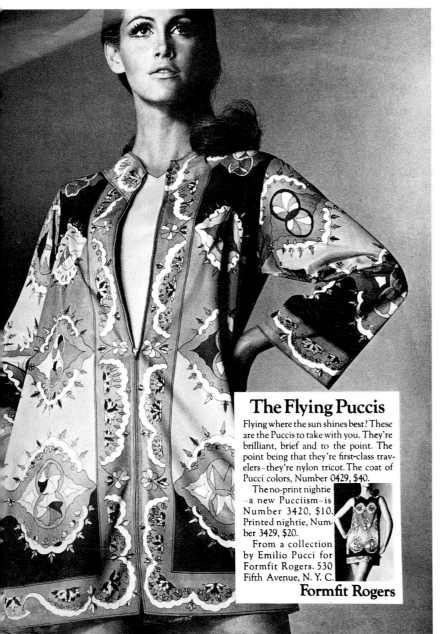

The Flying Puccis

Flying where the sun shines best? These are the Puccis to take with you. They're brilliant, brief and to the point. The point being that they're first-class travelers–they're nylon tricot. The coat of Pucci colors, Number 0429, $40.

The no-print nightie –a new Pucciism–is Number 3420, $10. Printed nightie, Number 3429, $20.

From a collection by Emilio Pucci for Formfit Rogers. 530 Fifth Avenue, N. Y. C.

Formfit Rogers

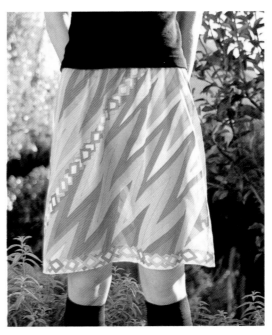

Advertisement for a nylon Pucci coat and a Pucci nightie that could easily serve as a dress today, from *Look*, November 26, 1968.

A Pucci half-slip, worn as a skirt. "Formfit Rogers."

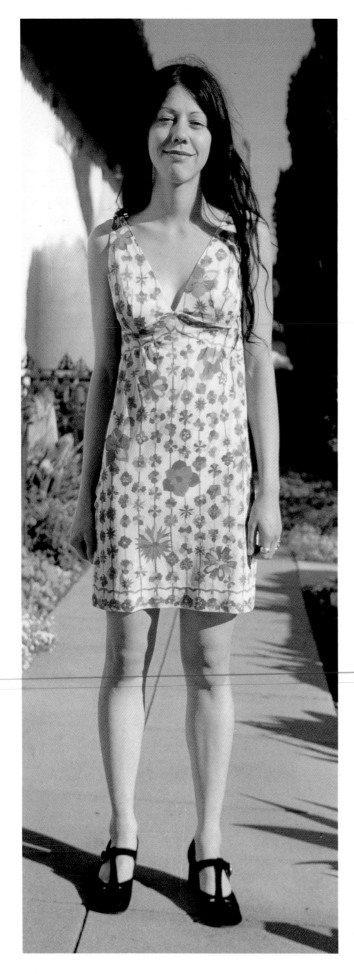

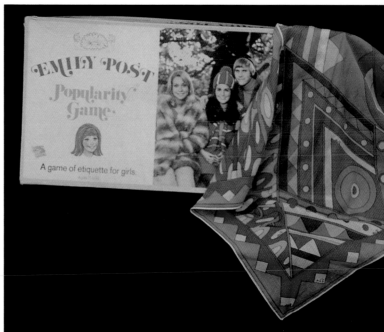

Two Pucci scarves.

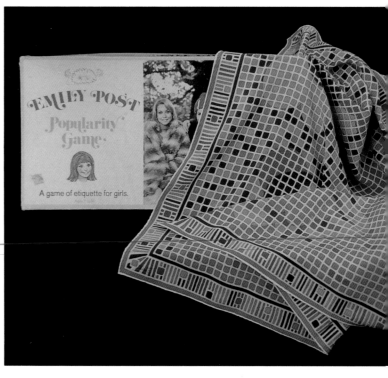

A Pucci nightie which Orion wears as a dress. "Formfit Rogers."

Oscar de la Renta

Known for romantic and opulent designs, Oscar de la Renta got his professional start in the 1950s in Spain, but was born in the Dominican Republic. By 1963, he had moved to New York where he continues to design under his own label; in 1997, he designed the gown which First Lady Hilary Clinton wore to the Presidential Inaugural Ball.

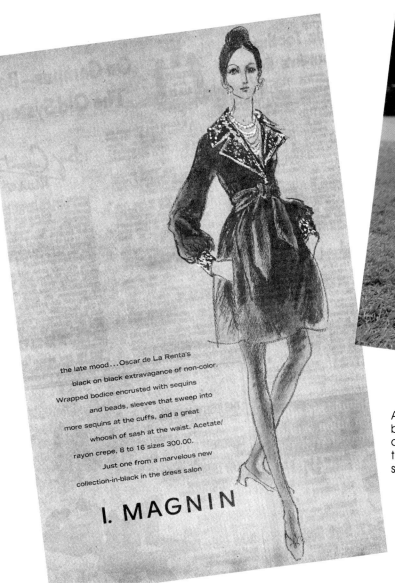

the late mood...Oscar de La Renta's black on black extravagance of non-color. Wrapped bodice encrusted with sequins and beads, sleeves that sweep into more sequins at the cuffs, and a great whoosh of sash at the waist. Acetate/ rayon crepe, 8 to 16 sizes 300.00.

Just one from a marvelous new collection-in-black in the dress salon

I. MAGNIN

Advertisement for an Oscar de la Renta dress from the *San Francisco Chronicle*, Monday, July 21, 1969. The headline of this edition read, "Men On Moon."

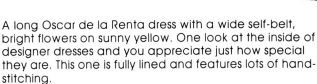

A long Oscar de la Renta dress with a wide self-belt, bright flowers on sunny yellow. One look at the inside of designer dresses and you appreciate just how special they are. This one is fully lined and features lots of hand-stitching.

Geoffrey Beene

Since he opened his own business in 1962, American designer Geoffrey Beene has designed chic, comfortable clothing for the active modern American woman. His deceptively simple styling emphasizes cut and line and has never gone out of style.

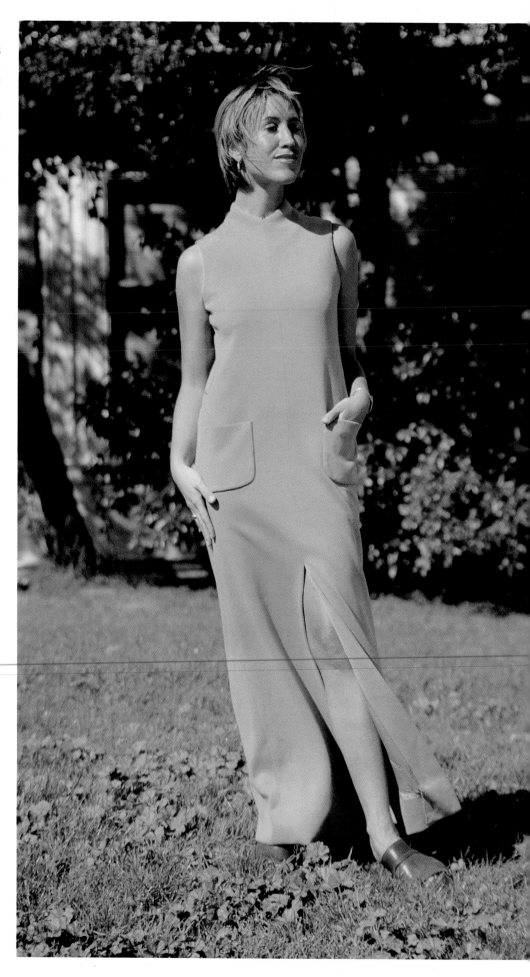

Long apple-green chavacette dress from the Geoffrey Beene boutique, at I. Magnin's, is fully lined in matching green taffeta, and is one of my favorites.

Diane Von Furstenberg

In 1969, Belgium-born Princess Diane Von Furstenburg moved to America. By 1971, she had opened a custom shop on New York's Fifth Avenue where she designed and sold moderately priced dresses of lightweight jersey made from patterns cut out on her dining room table. Her classic little midi-length styles, which she made until 1977, were affordable, comfortable, and fashionable. And yes, she really was royalty, by dint of her marriage to German Prince Egon Von Furstenberg!

Lilly Pulitzer

Lilly was not born a Pulitzer — she was married to a descendant of Joseph Pulitzer, the creator of the literary Pulitzer Prizes. She also never learned how to draft a pattern, but that didn't matter because her designs were so simple. Since 1960, her basic, brightly printed cotton shift, called "the Lilly," and other simple styles have been sold through her boutiques in resorts from Florida to Hawaii.

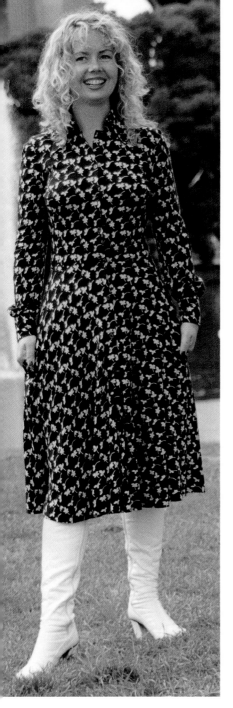

Graceful midi-length button-front dress by Diane Von Furstenberg, in her trademark dark print knit. The label says it's 100% acrylic, and that it was made in Italy.

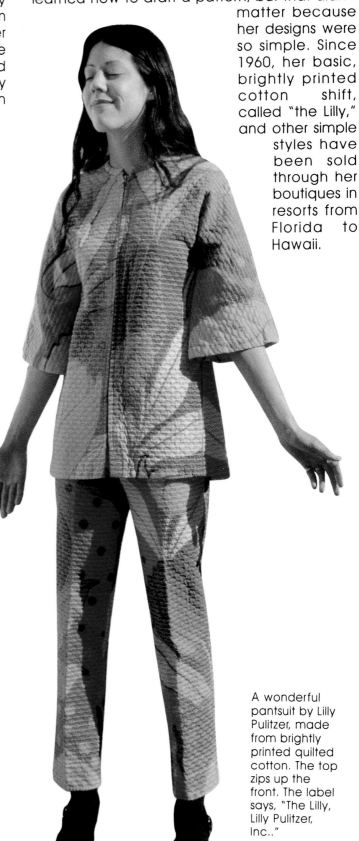

A wonderful pantsuit by Lilly Pulitzer, made from brightly printed quilted cotton. The top zips up the front. The label says, "The Lilly, Lilly Pulitzer, Inc.."

Chapter Thirteen

The New Romantics

The styles known as Romantic and neo-Victorian can be grouped with the retro styles, but two of the prominent companies of these nostalgic styles deserve a chapter to themselves: Gunne Sax and Arpeja.

Gunne Sax

American designer Jessica McClintock was taught to design clothes by her grandmother who was a seamstress and pattern maker; Jessica had designed her own clothes since she was a child. In 1969, she invested in a small company called Gunne Sax and built it into an American success story.

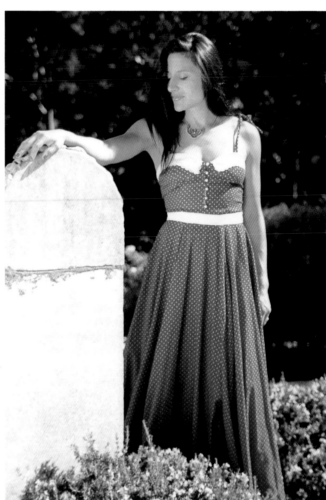

Red with white pindots, white satin trim and little pearl buttons down the bodice. Dress is 100% cotton, satin is 87% acetate and 13% nylon.

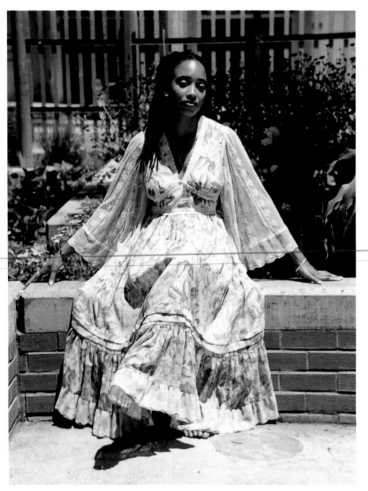

Pale yellow and gray print Gunne Sax with wide lace butterfly sleeves and ruffle. 65% polyester, 35% cotton.

During the '70s, many of the fashionable women owned at least one Gunne Sax dress or a dress in the Gunne Sax style manufactured by a competitor. You could spot a Gunne Sax immediately by its characteristic mix of calico, ruffles, ribbon and lace. Jessica McClintock even added lace to denim, and very successfully, too. Her day-length dresses went everywhere. Her long dresses were worn to weddings by brides, bridesmaids and mothers-of-the-bride, and to proms and Renaissance Faires. Often lacing up the front, and made from delicate, gauzy fabrics featuring Renaissance-inspired high waists and long, poetic sleeves, they made every woman wearing them look like Ophelia or Juliet.

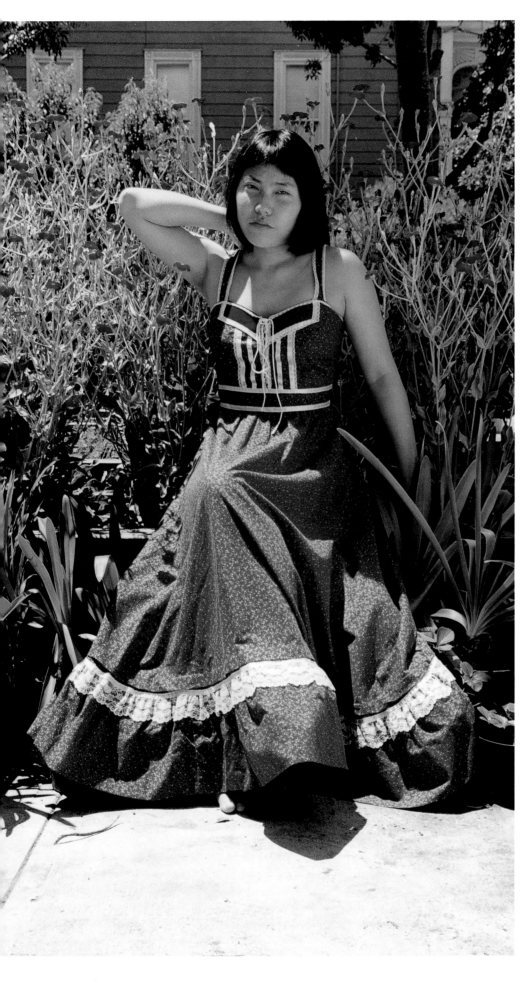

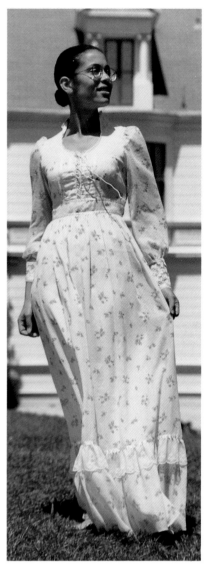

This beige voile Gunne Sax has faux seed pearls trimming the neckline, which rises high in back, giving it an Elizabethan look. It laces up the bodice, and features lace at the yoke, cuffs and trimming the skirt. 65% polyester, 35% cotton.

100% cotton, dark red calico trimmed with red velvet, white sating ribbon, and lace, laces up the bodice.

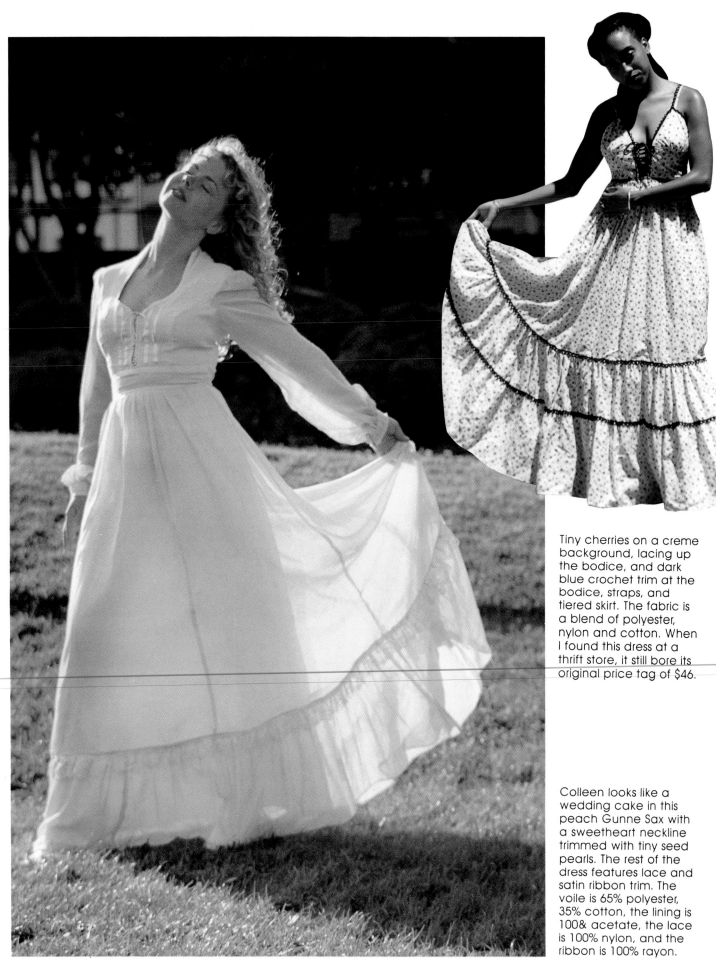

Tiny cherries on a creme background, lacing up the bodice, and dark blue crochet trim at the bodice, straps, and tiered skirt. The fabric is a blend of polyester, nylon and cotton. When I found this dress at a thrift store, it still bore its original price tag of $46.

Colleen looks like a wedding cake in this peach Gunne Sax with a sweetheart neckline trimmed with tiny seed pearls. The rest of the dress features lace and satin ribbon trim. The voile is 65% polyester, 35% cotton, the lining is 100& acetate, the lace is 100% nylon, and the ribbon is 100% rayon.

The Renaissance Faire

The first Renaissance Faire was held in Los Angeles in 1963 as a benefit for listener-sponsored radio station KPFK. The Faire, with colorful vendor booths and banners, strolling musicians, jousters, and jesters, was a taste of Olde England in California. The popular Southern California rock group The Byrds wrote a song about the Faire. By 1967, another Renaissance Faire was held in Northern California, and by 1976 there was a Faire in Minnesota. Gradually, Renaissance Faires were held also in other parts of the nation. It was more fun to attend the faires dressed in clothes that reflected the styles of the Renaissance.

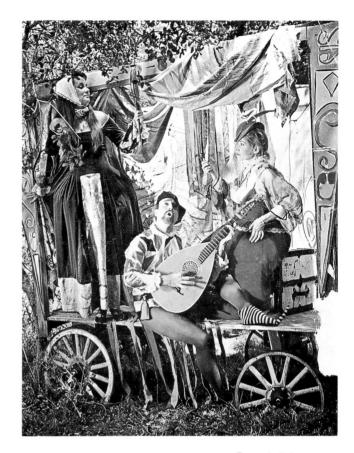

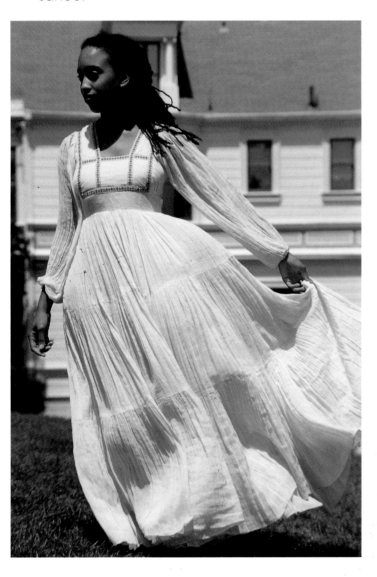

One of my favorites, and extremely Renaissance Faire in styling, this simple yet exquisite Gunne Sax features yards and yards of crinkly cotton in its three-tiered skirt and is trimmed only with embroidered ribbon.

From left to right, Phyllis Patterson, Ron Patterson, and Judith Kory, at the second Renaissance Faire, Los Angeles, 1964. Ron and Phyllis Patterson were the original creators and founders of the Renaissance Faire.

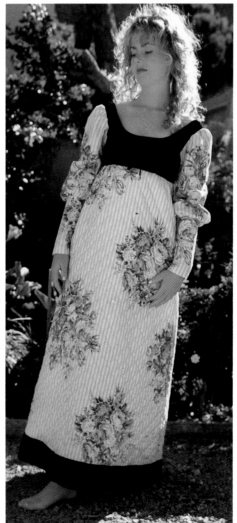

A Renaissance Faire-styled long dress by "Duchess Jr. loungewear", guaranteed to turn its wearer into Juliet or Ophelia. The black velvet bodice and band at the hem are rayon, the quilted skirt and romantic sleeves are 65% polyester and 35% cotton.

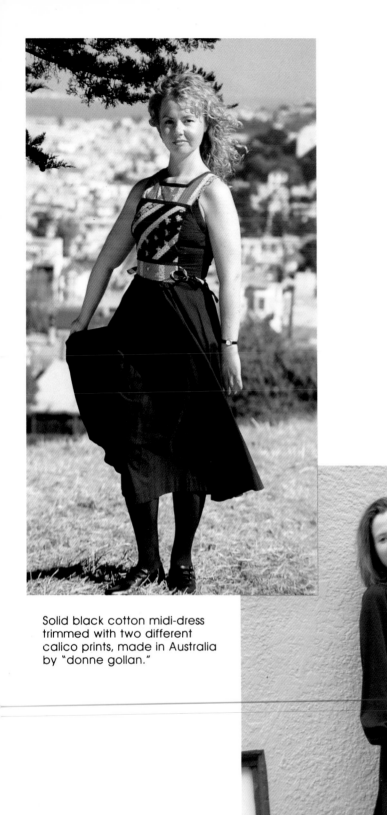

Solid black cotton midi-dress trimmed with two different calico prints, made in Australia by "donne gollan."

An unusually sophisticated Gunne Sax, with a graceful handkerchief hemline. Solid black trimmed with calico and narrow gold ribbons. The label says it's 50% polyester, 50% cotton, 87% acetate, and 13% nylon. Since that adds up to 200, the polyester and cotton is probably the black body of the dress, and the rest must be the trim.

Even if there hadn't been just enough of a label left in the dress, I would still have recognized this as Gunne Sax, due to the distinctive features like red satin ribbon, black lace, and black calico trim.

Arpeja

The prettiness of clothing made under the Arpeja labels added significantly to the romanitc style of the late '60s and early '70s. Arpeja produced moderately priced fashions every bit as poetic as the Gunne Sax clothing but less like a costume and more suitable for everyday wear. The Arpeja line had two labels: Young Innocent and Young Edwardian. The clothes are '30s retro in style and exceptionally romantic.

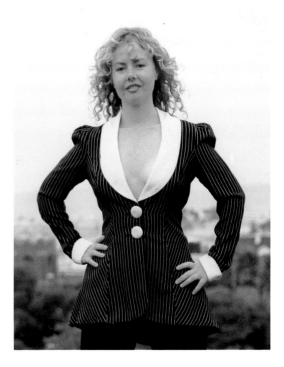

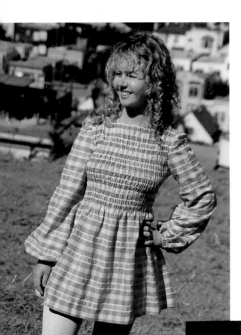

Very low-cut pinstriped crepe jacket probably originally came with matching wide pants. It's trimmed with satin shawl collar and cuffs, and big white satin buttons, and it features small shoulder pads. "Young Edwardian, by Arpeja."

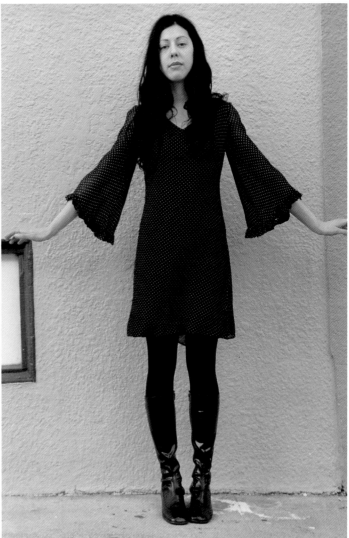

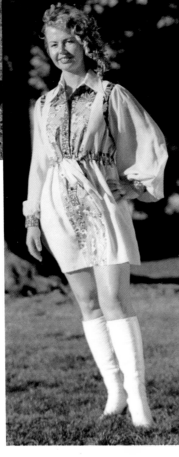

Cute as a button woven blue gingham dress, aptly labeled, "Young Innocent, by Arpeja", has an elasticized bodice.

The body of this charming mini is eggshell-colored voile, and it's trimmed with three different calico prints. "Young Edwardian, by Arpeja."

White pindots on black silk chiffon. The floaty sleeves end in ruffles. "Young Edwardian, by Arpeja."

$\mathcal{A}$ Hazy Shade of Winter

Women froze their legs during the first few mini-coat winters until they switched to midi- and maxi-coats. These ankle-length coats opened to reveal lots of leg, giving a cute "flasher" effect.

Fabulous fakes

By the mid-'60s, a rage for antique fur coats had swept the country and warehouses specializing in antique furs could be found in most major cities. The widespread wearing of antique furs continued throughout the '70s and even into the '80s until the influence of animal rights and anti-fur movements changed popular thinking. Some of the fashionable women who used to wear antique furs reasoned that the coats were so old that the animals would have died of old age, anyway. Today, most vintage stores don't carry antique furs.

An acceptable alternative to wearing real fur was provided in fake furs, some of which were just as warm as the real fur. Fake furs were made from — what else? — polyester. By the mid-'60s, even the most ardent fur-wearer felt a bit reluctant to wear the fur of the exquisite and endangered leopards, but imitations of those beautiful animals were readily available and much more affordable, too. Sometimes fake furs were mixed with leather for a furry version of the popular patchwork effect.

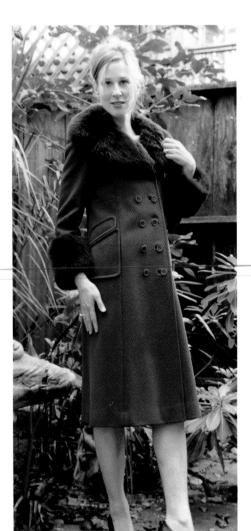

Burgundy wool midi-length coat with fake fur trim. "Pina de Roma."

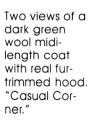

Two views of a dark green wool midi-length coat with real fur-trimmed hood. "Casual Corner."

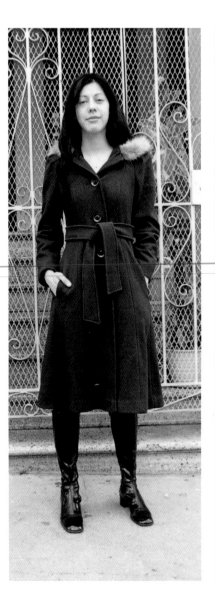

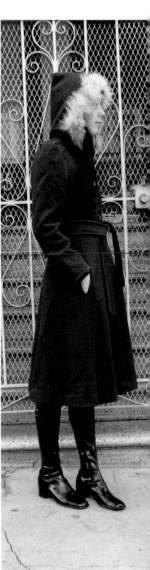

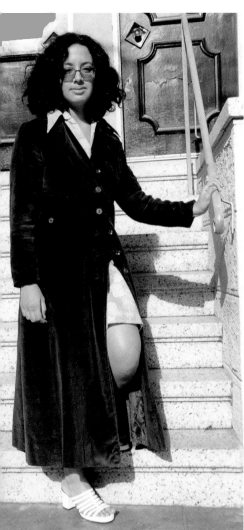

Beautiful dark green plush maxi-length coat.

Labels on pleather jackets will tell you not to dry clean them, but to just wipe them with a damp cloth to get off surface dirt. This may be fine for simple surface dirt, but I've discovered that when the lining is dirty, or the pleather needs more than just wiping down, you can throw them in the washing machine. Wash in cold water, and for goodness sake, don't put them in the dryer! Instead, take the jacket out as soon as the wash cycle is over and hang it up to dry. And you do know better than to try ironing them, don't you?

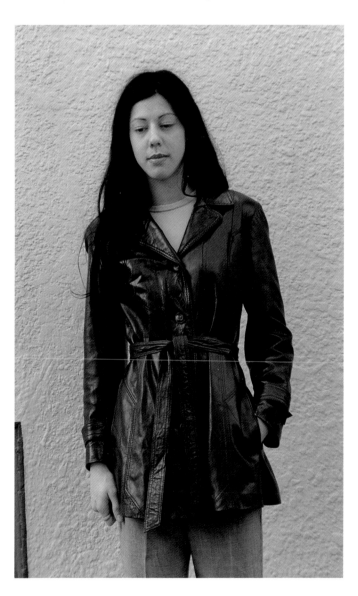

Classic belted brown leather jacket. No label.

Leather and Pleather

All leather jackets have never really gone out of fashion. During the mid- to late '60s and early '70s, a patchwork effect was carried out in leather in various styles. The cleverest and most desirable leather patchwork is the look of scales, where differently colored leather is sewn together to form a jacket that seems to have been made from the skin of some exotic, rainbow colored fish.

Another '60s leather look is the classic fringed suede jacket, which will be forever associated with hippies. Good fringed jackets have deep fringes in interesting patterns and the very best include decorative beads.

Vinyl jackets, popularly known as "pleather" (for plastic leather), may have once been merely a cheap substitute for leather, but they deserve a special classification of their own. The best ones don't even attempt to look like leather, but are made in colors nature never dreamed of: pastels and whites. Don't look for warmth in a "pleather" jacket; they're not as warm as leather. Do look for a light jacket that is quite simply fun to wear.

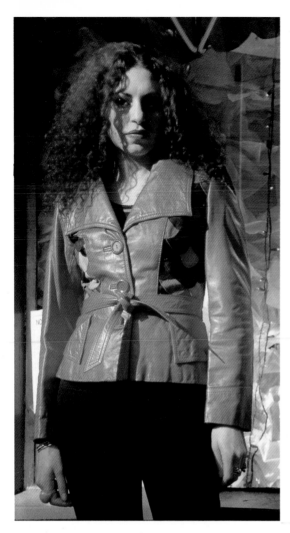

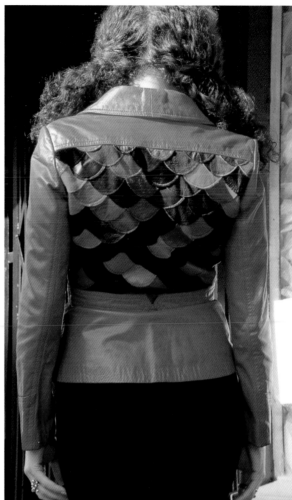

Front and back
views of leather
jacket deco-
rated with multi-
colored leather
"scales."
Courtesy Martini
Mercantile.

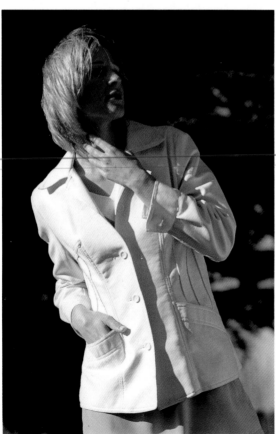

Denim-colored suede double-
breasted mini-coat or jacket.

White pleather jacket.

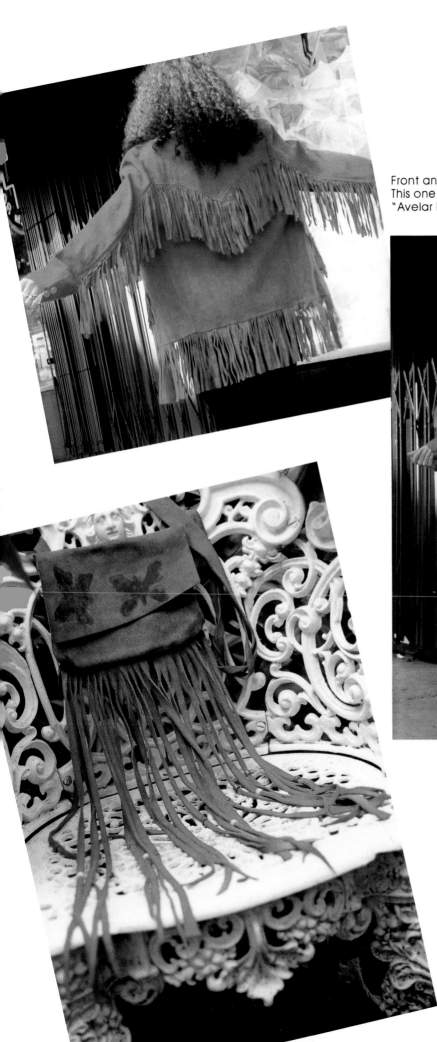

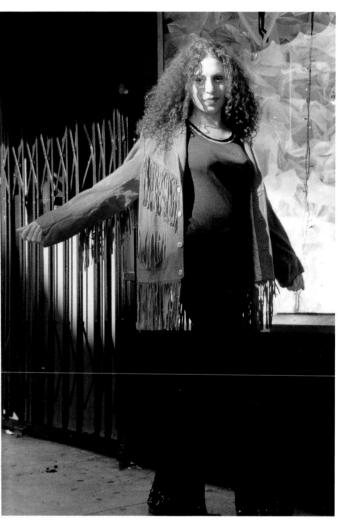

Front and back views of a classic fringed suede jacket. This one was made in Mexico for "Avelar Productions." Courtesy Martini Mercantile.

Fringed and beaded suede shoulder-bag with stenciled butterflies on the flap.

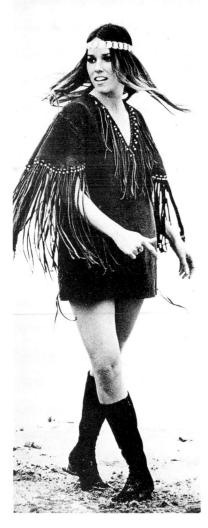

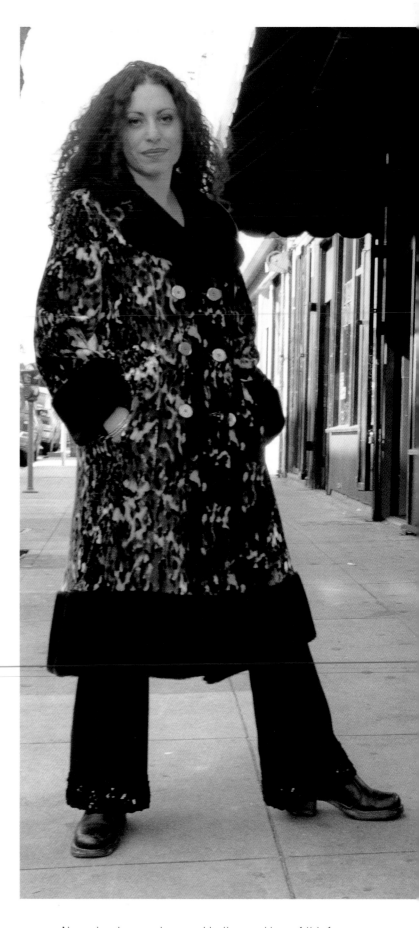

Actress Barbara Hershey in fringed and beaded leather, from *Show*, 1970.

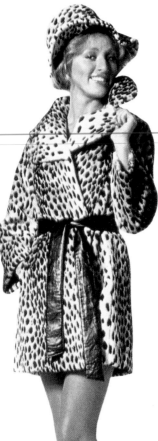

A faux leopard mini-coat from the *Frederick's of Hollywood* catalogue, 1978.

No animals were harmed in the making of this faux leopard midi-length coat. Courtesy Martini Mercantile.

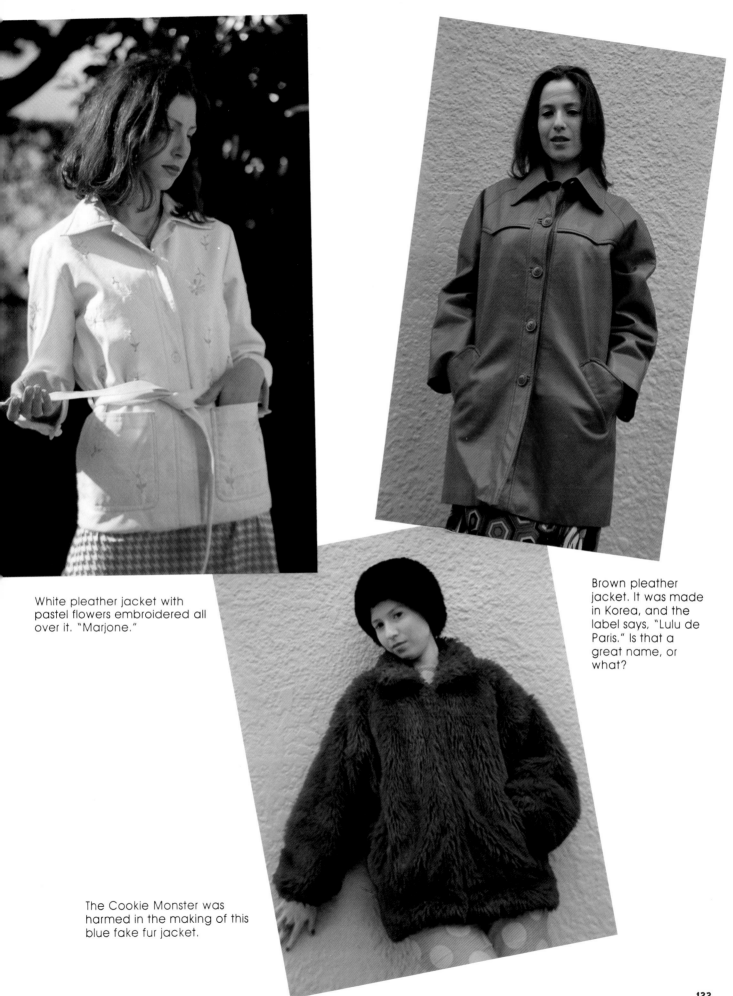

White pleather jacket with pastel flowers embroidered all over it. "Marjone."

Brown pleather jacket. It was made in Korea, and the label says, "Lulu de Paris." Is that a great name, or what?

The Cookie Monster was harmed in the making of this blue fake fur jacket.

133

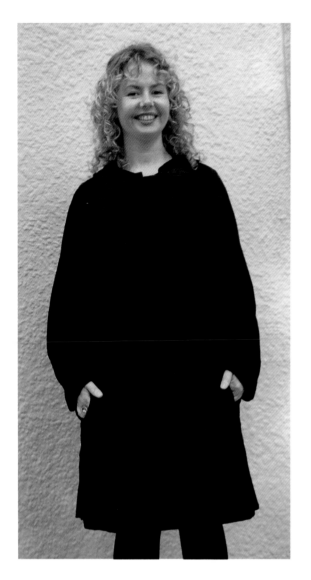

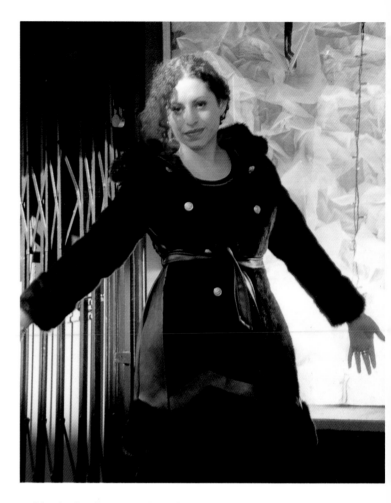

Black pleather and fake fur mini-coat. Courtesy Martini Mercantile.

Double breasted faux pony mini-length coat.

The Velvet Blazer

Velvet blazers, worn throughout the '70s, have never gone out of fashion. They are classic in styling, no matter how many buttons they may feature. Made in every solid color velvet, they were also made in velvet prints, and those are some of the best.

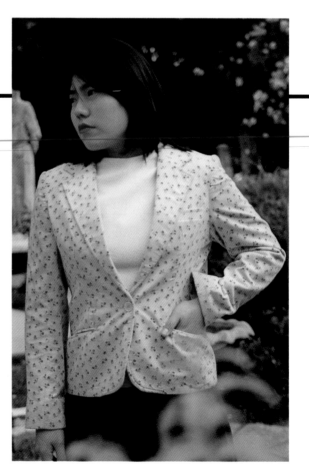

Velvet jacket has little flowers on a creme background. "Falcone."

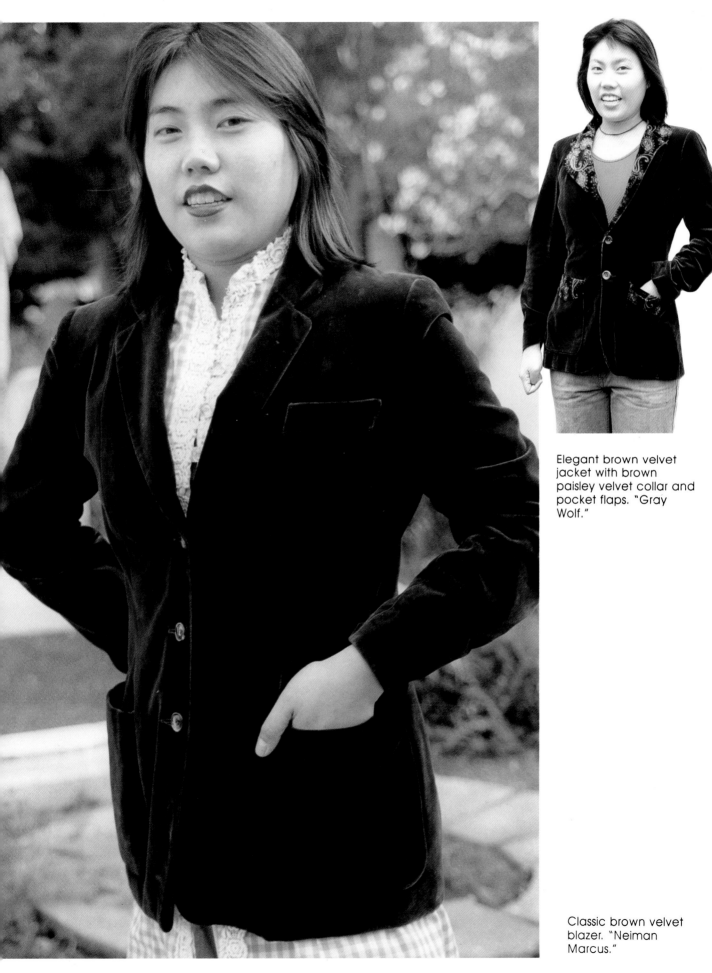

Elegant brown velvet jacket with brown paisley velvet collar and pocket flaps. "Gray Wolf."

Classic brown velvet blazer. "Neiman Marcus."

135

Chapter Fifteen

These Boots Are Made For Walkin'

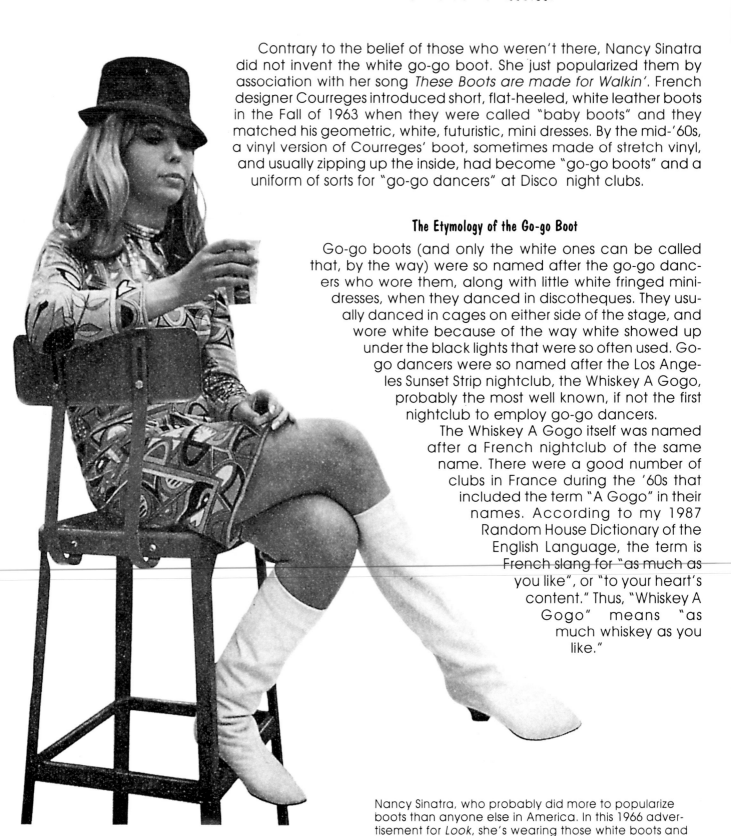

Contrary to the belief of those who weren't there, Nancy Sinatra did not invent the white go-go boot. She just popularized them by association with her song *These Boots are made for Walkin'*. French designer Courreges introduced short, flat-heeled, white leather boots in the Fall of 1963 when they were called "baby boots" and they matched his geometric, white, futuristic, mini dresses. By the mid-'60s, a vinyl version of Courreges' boot, sometimes made of stretch vinyl, and usually zipping up the inside, had become "go-go boots" and a uniform of sorts for "go-go dancers" at Disco night clubs.

The Etymology of the Go-go Boot

Go-go boots (and only the white ones can be called that, by the way) were so named after the go-go dancers who wore them, along with little white fringed mini-dresses, when they danced in discotheques. They usually danced in cages on either side of the stage, and wore white because of the way white showed up under the black lights that were so often used. Go-go dancers were so named after the Los Angeles Sunset Strip nightclub, the Whiskey A Gogo, probably the most well known, if not the first nightclub to employ go-go dancers.

The Whiskey A Gogo itself was named after a French nightclub of the same name. There were a good number of clubs in France during the '60s that included the term "A Gogo" in their names. According to my 1987 Random House Dictionary of the English Language, the term is French slang for "as much as you like", or "to your heart's content." Thus, "Whiskey A Gogo" means "as much whiskey as you like."

Nancy Sinatra, who probably did more to popularize boots than anyone else in America. In this 1966 advertisement for *Look*, she's wearing those white boots and what looks like a Pucci dress.

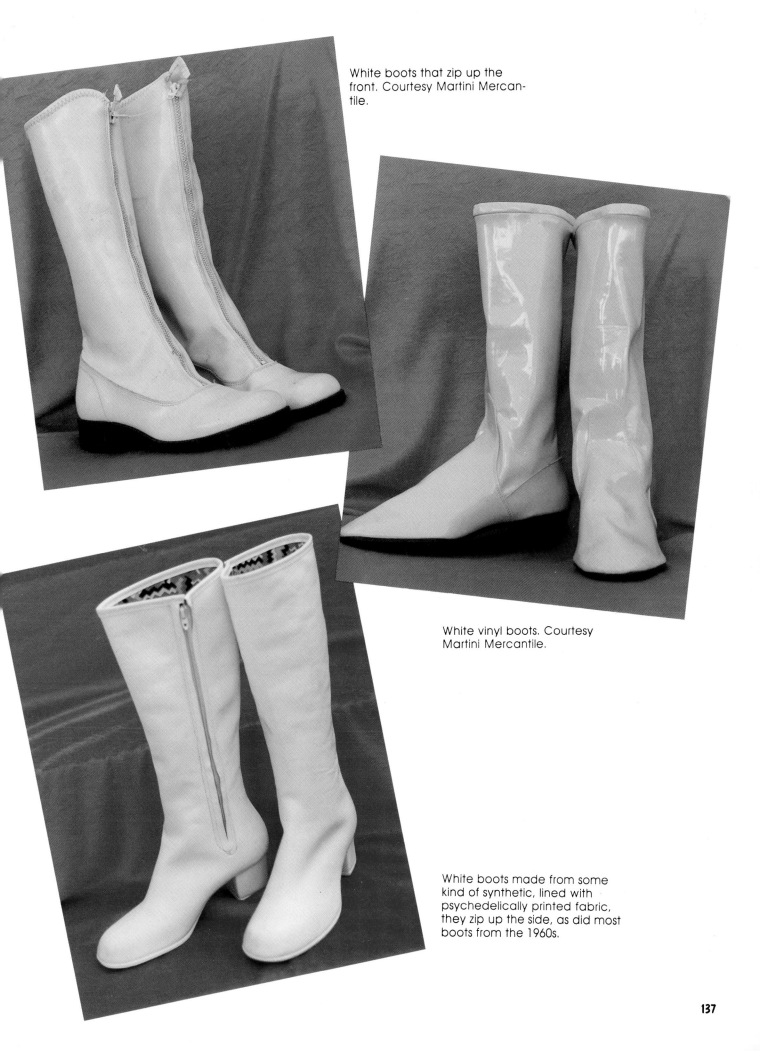

White boots that zip up the front. Courtesy Martini Mercantile.

White vinyl boots. Courtesy Martini Mercantile.

White boots made from some kind of synthetic, lined with psychedelically printed fabric, they zip up the side, as did most boots from the 1960s.

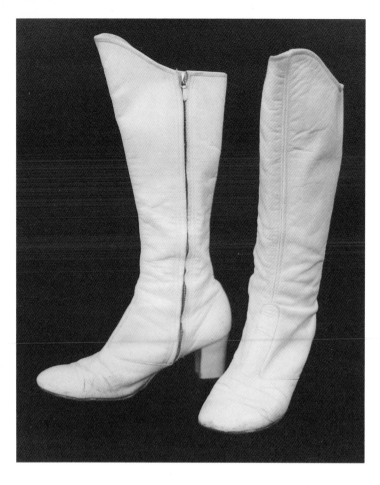

White cowgirl-styled leather boots.

Classic white vinyl, side-zipped boots.

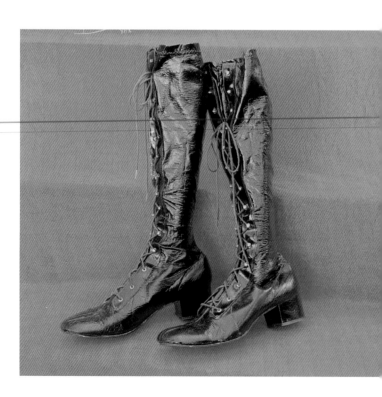

Black vinyl and tapestry boots with an interesting heel.
Courtesy Martini Mercantile.

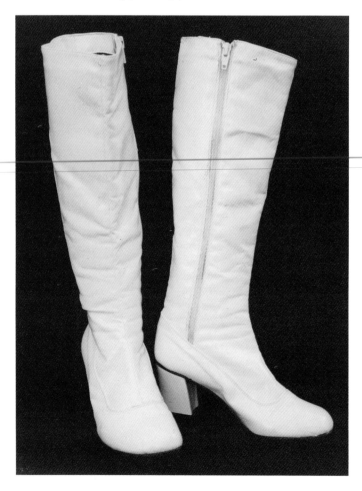

Brown stretch vinyl boots lace up the front.

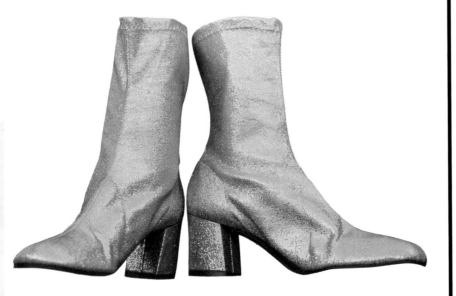

Gold lame stretch "Beatle boots." Courtesy Martini Mercantile

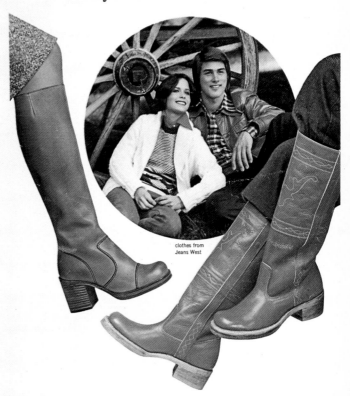
Brown vinyl side-zipped boots with decorative brass buckles.

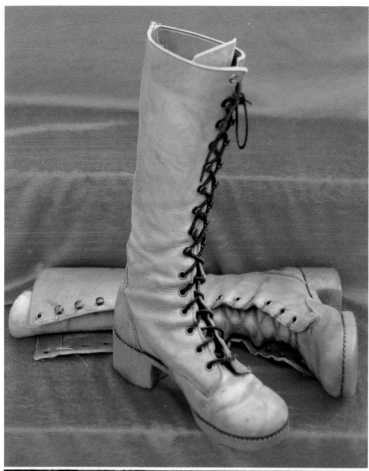

Platform Shoes

Hard to believe, but the platform shoe really had a life span of only about four years, five years tops. By 1969, the hippest shoes featured a very small platform sole. As the early '70s progressed, the platform grew bigger, to finally culminate in the thickest platforms we so avidly collect today. At their highest and best, platforms are almost a kind of shoe sculpture, appropriate for display on a tabletop.

A Warning: balancing on the really high platforms can be a problem, and quite a few women have fallen from them, sometimes to the tune of a broken ankle. Walk carefully!

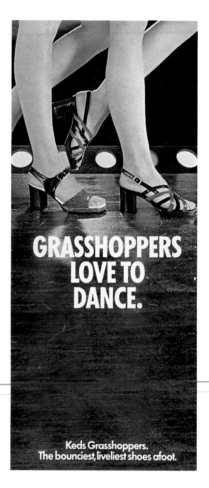

GRASSHOPPERS LOVE TO DANCE.

Keds Grasshoppers.
The bounciest, liveliest shoes afoot.

Advertisement for modified platform shoes, from *Woman's Day*, May, 1974.

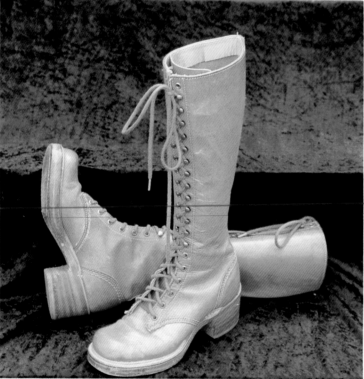

Two pairs of Frye"-style boots, both lacing up the front.

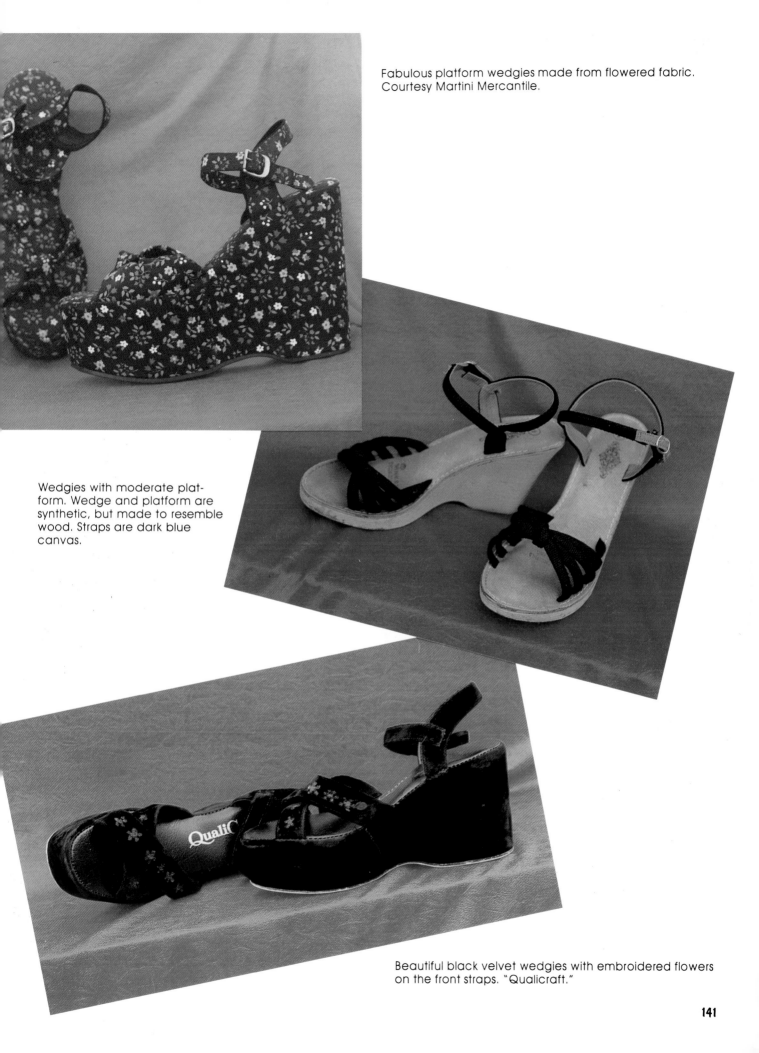

Fabulous platform wedgies made from flowered fabric.
Courtesy Martini Mercantile.

Wedgies with moderate platform. Wedge and platform are
synthetic, but made to resemble
wood. Straps are dark blue
canvas.

Beautiful black velvet wedgies with embroidered flowers
on the front straps. "Qualicraft."

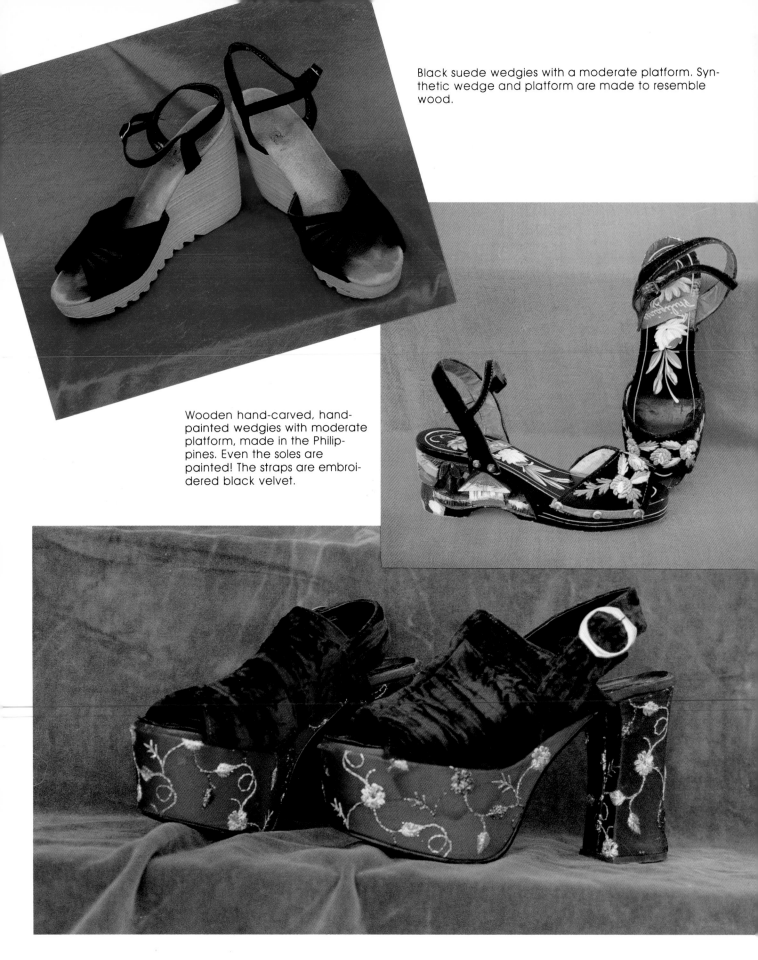

Black suede wedgies with a moderate platform. Synthetic wedge and platform are made to resemble wood.

Wooden hand-carved, hand-painted wedgies with moderate platform, made in the Philippines. Even the soles are painted! The straps are embroidered black velvet.

Gorgeous maroon platforms. The heels and high platforms are covered with maroon satin, embroidered in silver, the front and straps are maroon crushed velvet.

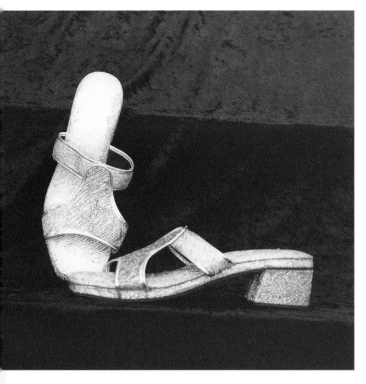

Gold lame sandals with a moderate platform and chunky pyramid-heels.

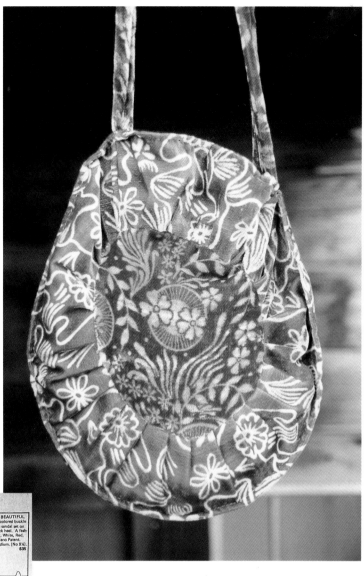

Brown velvet shoulderbag with white flower designs, in a kind of batik effect.

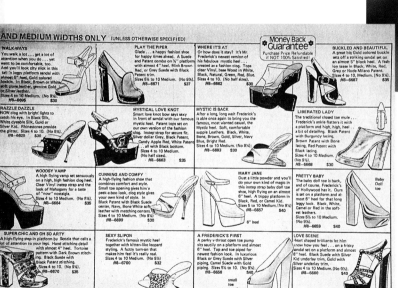

A whole page of extreme platform shoes from the 1973 *Frederick's of Hollywood* catalogue.

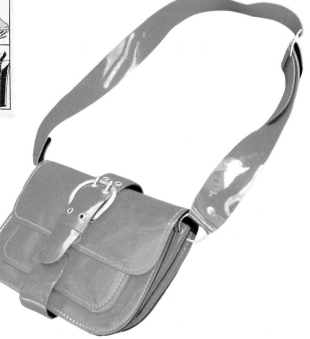

Hot pink patent leather shoulderbag.

Chapter Sixteen
You Can Make It If You Try

Want a swirl skirt, but can't find one? Want a fake leopard mini-coat, but they cost too much in the vintage shops? Or, you've been to the flea markets, the thrift shops, and the vintage shops, you've waded through miles of polyester, but there's one dress — a paisley polyester mini that you found in the pages of a 1968 copy of *Harper's Bazaar*—it's the cutest little thing in the world, and you can't find it anywhere. Never fear! If you have a sewing machine and you know how to use it, you can always recreate vintage clothing from any period, providing, of course, that you can find the pattern. Sewing patterns from the '50s and before are harder, though in no way impossible, to find, and might run you into some money. But patterns from the '60s and '70s are still comparatively easy to find in thrift shops or garage sales, and cost anywhere from mere pennies to a few dollars.

During the '70s, Butterick patterns even published a line called Young Designer, which included designers like Betsey Johnson, Kenzo, and Margit Brandt, of Copenhagen. Old Betsey Johnson patterns are always in style.

A word of warning: don't try to judge the year of a particular fashion's origin by the copyright dates on pattern envelopes. With the possible exception of Vogue patterns, American pattern companies seem to wait a few years to make sure a particular style is successful before issuing a pattern for it, so the patterns they sell are never at the cutting edge; they tend to be just a little out of date.

Now that you've found your pattern, you need fabric from the period, although you can make up some great vintage patterns using contemporary fabric. Vintage fabric may be a little harder to find, but it's still do-able. Try flea markets, garage and estate sales. Older women who used to sew may have decided to finally clear out their sewing rooms. I found much of the fabric in my collection at the estate sale of a woman who had been a dressmaker. Her patterns were a disappointment — she had very conservative taste in clothes — but her psychedelic and retro print polyesters were top notch.

Hopefully, matching the right fabrics with the right pattern will be obvious. You wouldn't take that psychedelic, pop art doubleknit, printed all over with peace signs, and turn it into a granny dress, when it's obviously meant to become bellbottoms, right? Or the dark green polyester with little Flappers printed on it — can you say retro? And that great Hawaiian print on polished cotton can be turned into a long holoku, if there's enough yardage; if not, how about a classic shift?

Speaking of enough yardage, sometimes you might find a mere yard of fabric, but you just love the print. How to use it? Check the pages of this book for examples of prints mixed with solids. A word of advice about sewing polyesters: you'll need a special needle, something called a ball-point. Don't panic, you can find ball-point needles wherever sewing supplies are sold. Otherwise, you'll find your machine producing some of the weirdest, most irregular stitches you've ever seen. You can use any kind of thread, within reason: nylon, cotton, silk, or cotton-wrapped polyester.

Oppostie page: Betsey Johnson designs by Butterick. In looking for designer patterns like these, it makes no difference if the envelope is in bad shape (Unless it's intended for framing!). What's important is making sure all the pattern pieces are there.

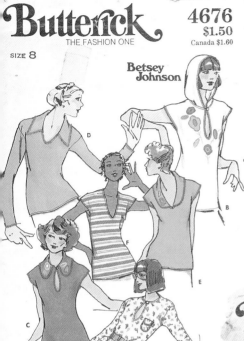

Butterick THE FASHION ONE
4676
$1.50
Canada $1.60

SIZE 8

Betsey Johnson

SIZED FOR **MODERATE STRETCH** KNITS ONLY
SEE **SELECT-A-KNIT** GAUGE ON ENVELOPE BACK

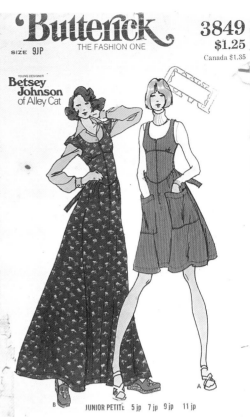

Butterick THE FASHION ONE
3849
$1.25
Canada $1.35

SIZE 9JP

YOUNG DESIGNER
Betsey Johnson of Alley Cat

JUNIOR PETITE 5 jp 7 jp 9 jp 11 jp

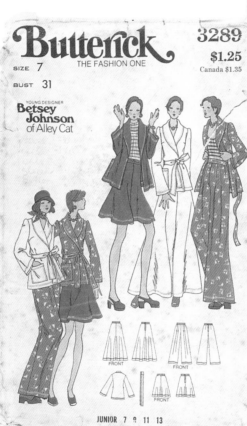

Butterick THE FASHION ONE
3289
$1.25
Canada $1.35

SIZE 7
BUST 31

YOUNG DESIGNER
Betsey Johnson of Alley Cat

FRONT   FRONT

FRONT

JUNIOR 7 9 11 13

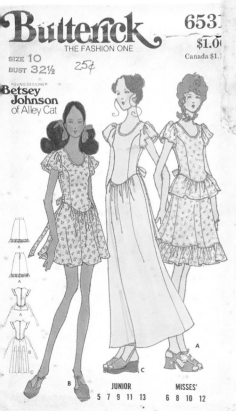

Butterick THE FASHION ONE
653
$1.00
Canada $1.1

SIZE 10
BUST 32½   25¢

Betsey Johnson of Alley Cat

JUNIOR
5 7 9 11 13

MISSES'
6 8 10 12

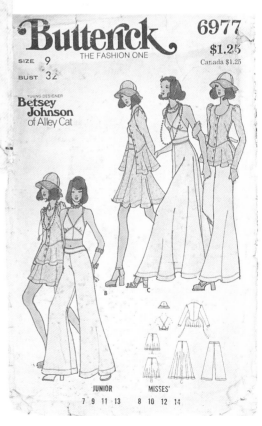

Butterick THE FASHION ONE
6977
$1.25
Canada $1.25

SIZE 9
BUST 32

YOUNG DESIGNER
Betsey Johnson of Alley Cat

JUNIOR
7 9 11 13

MISSES'
8 10 12 14

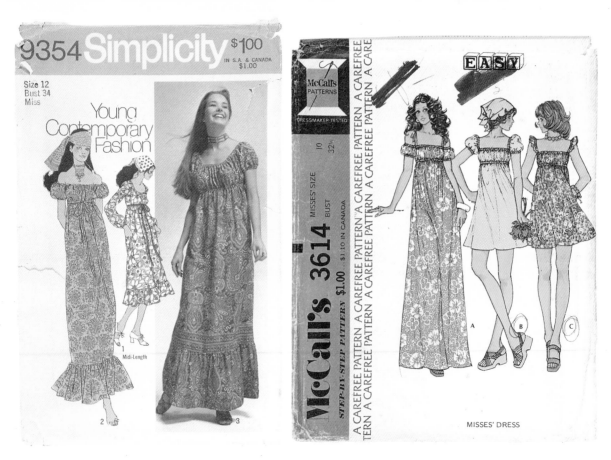

Patterns for empire dresses, from Simplicity and McCall's. The Simplicity pattern is from 1971, and the McCall's is from 1973.

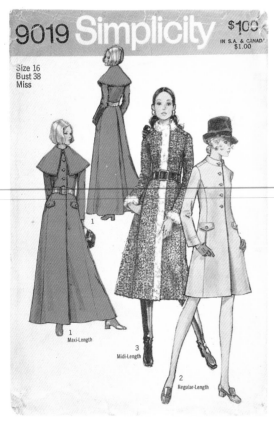

Simplicity pattern for a coat in midi and maxi-length, from 1970.

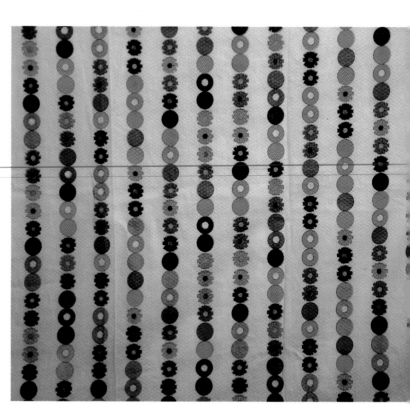

Lines of daisies and what looks like lifesavers in green and pink on white pique, perfect for a simple shift.

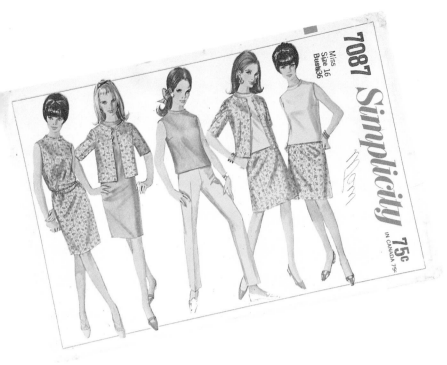

Simplicity pattern from 1967, for basic a Jackie Kennedy-type wardrobe.

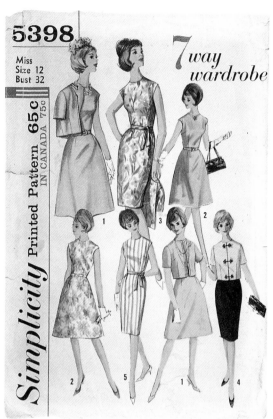

An entire Jackie Kennedy-type wardrobe from 1964, by Simplicity.

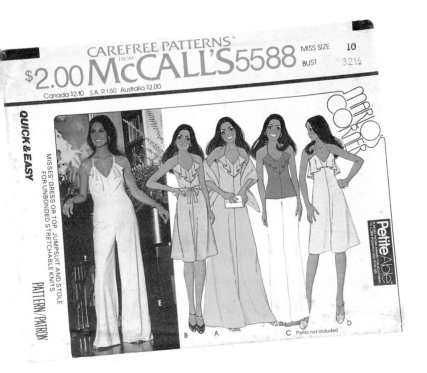

Marlo Thomas models a jumpsuit for "Marlo's Corner", McCall's, 1977.

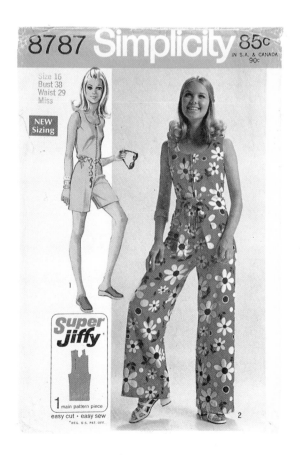

A jumpsuit from 1970, by Simplicity.

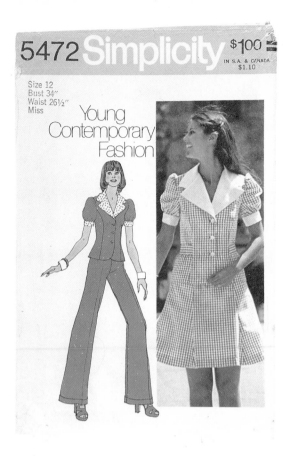

A retro pantsuit from Simplicity, 1972.

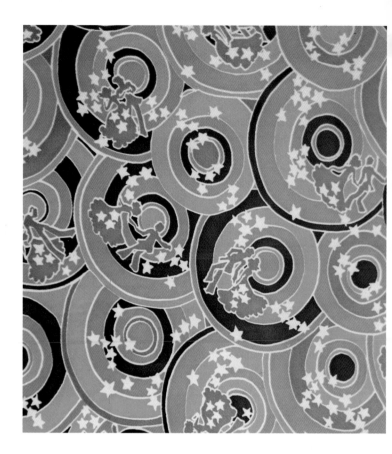

Retro print on polyester jersey. Surrounded by stars, an art deco couple dances amidst gold, blue and black swirls.

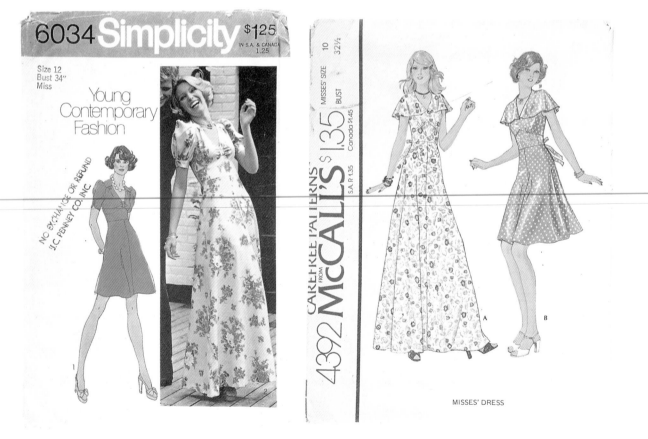

Patterns for retro designs that look great as either short or long dresses, by Simplicity and McCall's. The Simplicity pattern is from 1973, the McCall's from 1975.

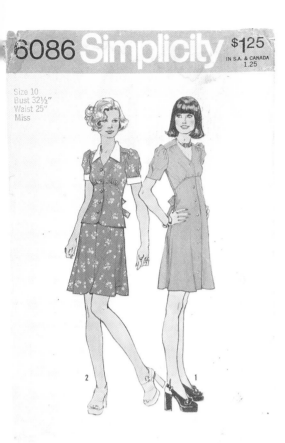

6086 Simplicity $125
IN S.A. & CANADA
1.25

Size 10
Bust 32½"
Waist 25"
Miss

Retro pattern by Simplicity for a
dress or suit, from 1973.

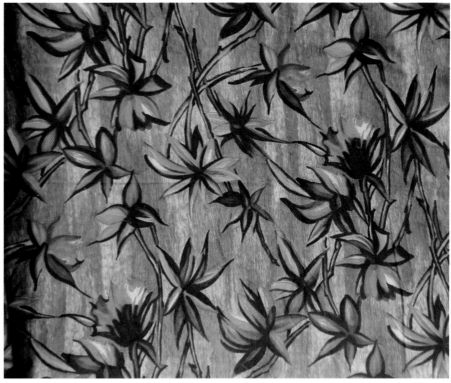

Glowing orange flowers on green decorate this Hawaiian cotton fabric.

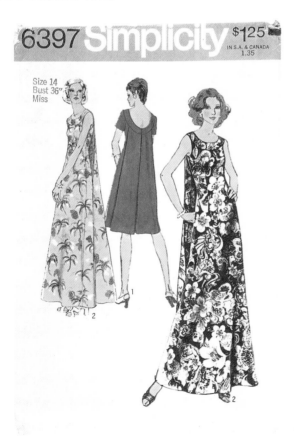

6397 Simplicity $125
IN S.A. & CANADA
1.35

Size 14
Bust 36"
Miss

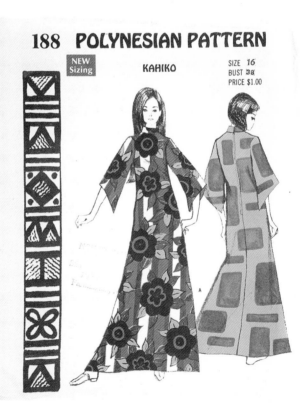

188 POLYNESIAN PATTERN

NEW Sizing

KAHIKO

SIZE 16
BUST 38
PRICE $1.00

Two patterns for Hawaiian dresses. The Simplicity pattern
is from 1974, the Polynesian Pattern is not dated.

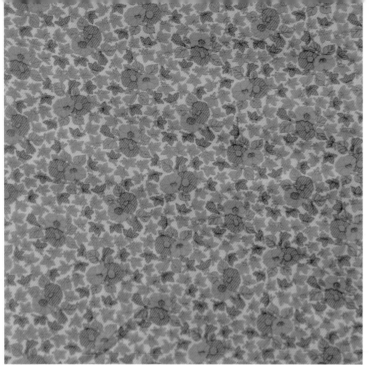

Bright pink and turquoise flowers on green challis

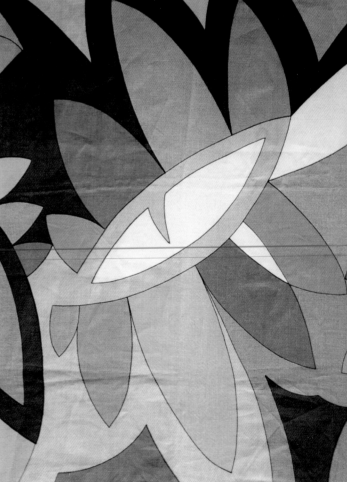

Bright flowers on dark green cotton. The selvage says, "VHY Hawaiian textiles #619."

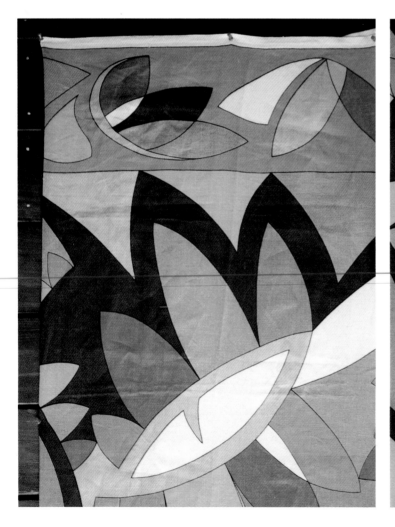

Two views of a linen-look fabric featuring humongous purple, lavender and blue flowers and a border design.

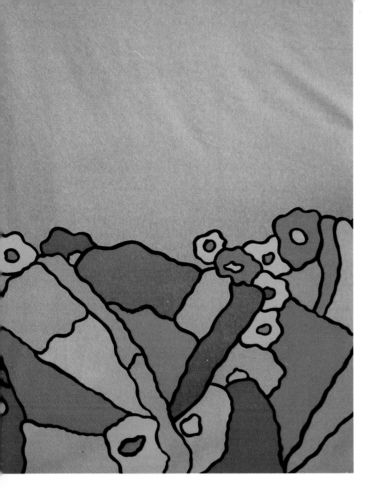
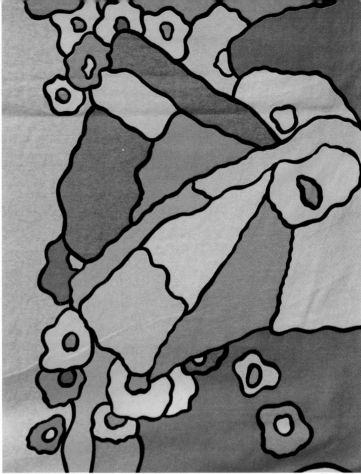

Two views of a blue cotton jersey fabric with a bright, Peter Max-inspired, border print. The selvage says, "Birchwood Fabrics, Inc.."

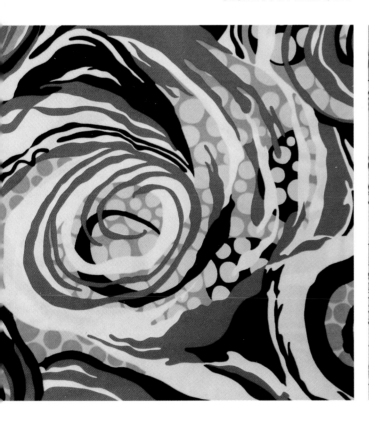

Red, white, and blue swirls on polkadots decorate heavy stretch polyester.

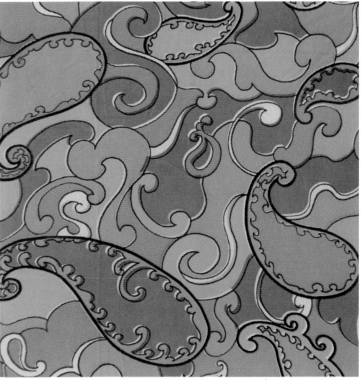

Polyester jersey printed with psychedelic pink, turquoise and green paisleys.

Chapter Seventeen
Charlie's Angels

Just as Jacqueline Kennedy's proper, ladylike demeanor symbolizes the early '60s, Farrah Fawcett's take-charge feminism symbolizes the late '70s. Farrah played the role of a detective on the television hit show "Charlie's Angels." She and her two show sisters could solve a murder and fill out a mean bikini with equal ease. Beauty salons everywhere blow-dried their clients' hair to resemble Farrah's famous breezy locks. And these TV characters really wore the pants — in the form of jumpsuits and pants suits, bellbottomed of course!

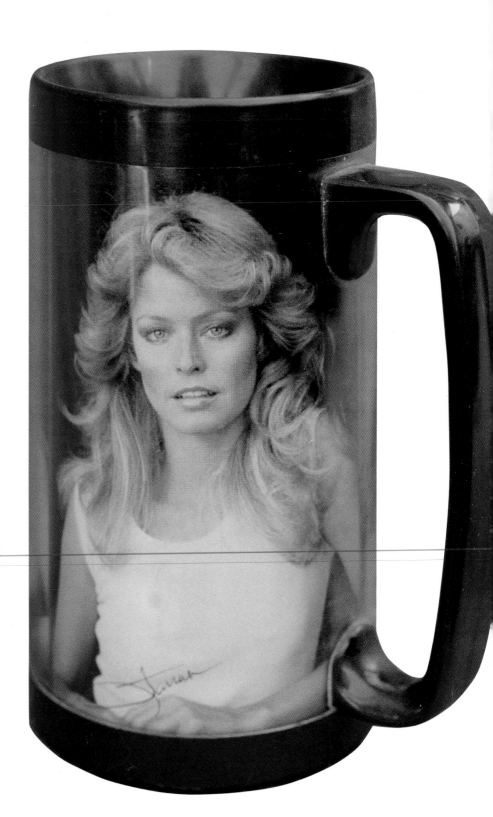

Farrah Fawcett on a plastic mug. "Thermo-Serv", made in USA.

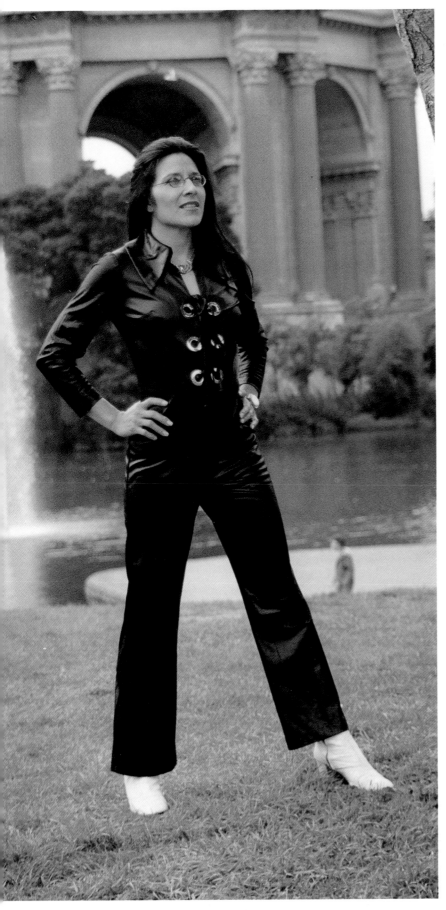

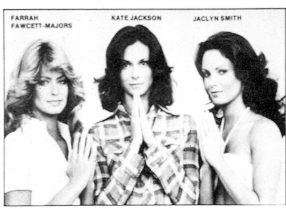

All three of Charlie's Angels, from *Photoplay*, February, 1977.

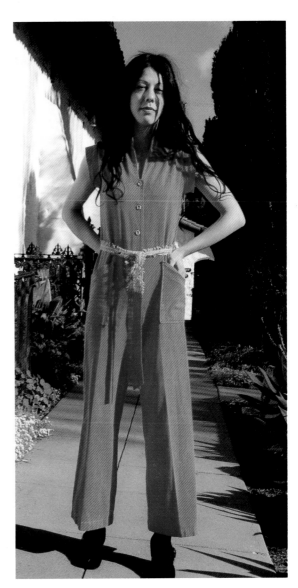

Jumpsuit made from some nameless shiny black stretch synthetic laces up the front, with outsize brass grommets. No label.

Brick colored cotton jumpsuit ties at the waist with macramé jute belt and buttons down the front with bone buttons. "Byer, California."

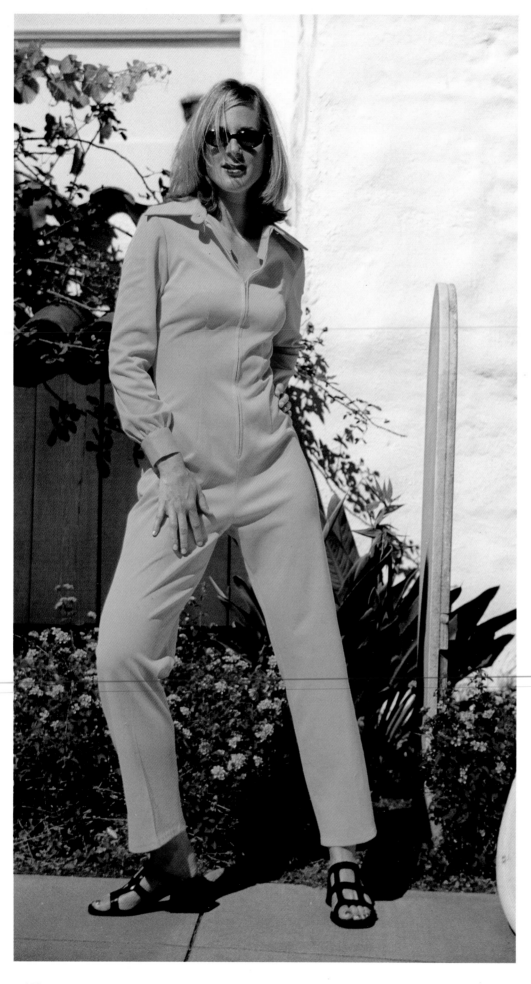

Bright yellow double-knit polyester jumpsuit sips up the front. "Krist."

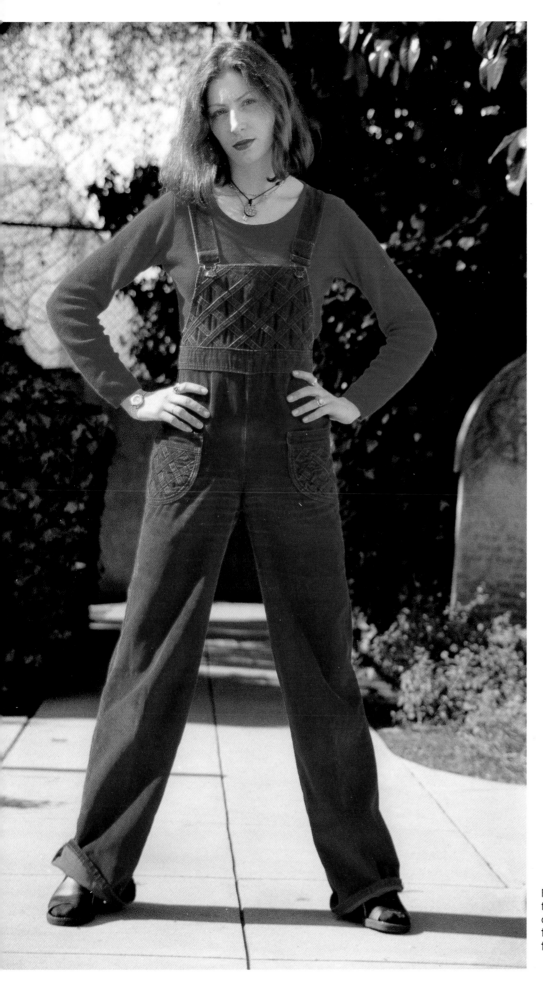

Rust colored corduroy overalls
feature latticework on the bib
and pockets. Casey is wearing
the pants really long, the way
they were worn in the 1970s.

Pantsuits

The double-knit pantsuit has become permanently associated with the '70s. It truly is so hideous that it's beautiful — I can say no more.

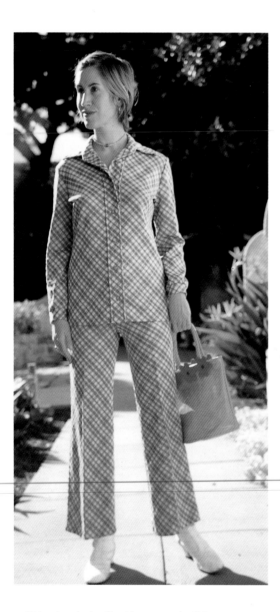

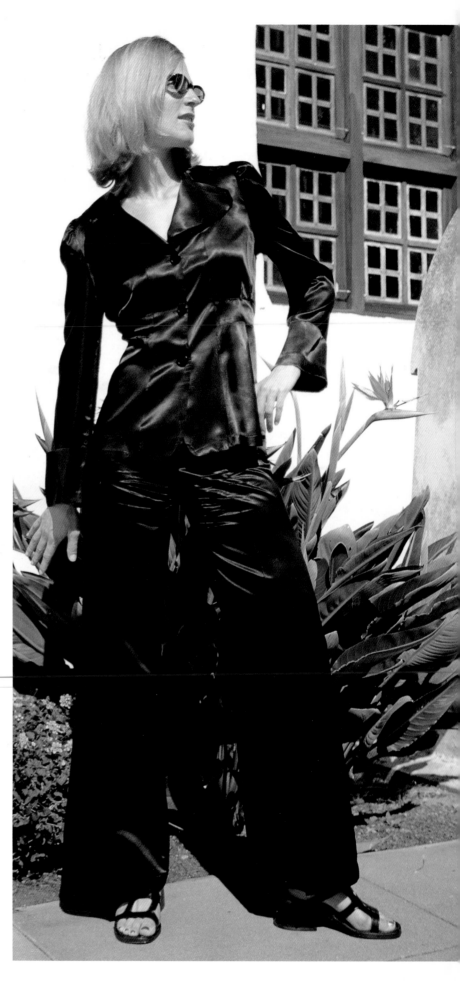

This classic bellbottom pantsuit is brown on beige checked double-knit. The label says, "Stage 7", and informs us that it's 55% polyester, 45% acetate.

Black satin pantsuit with very wide legs. No label.

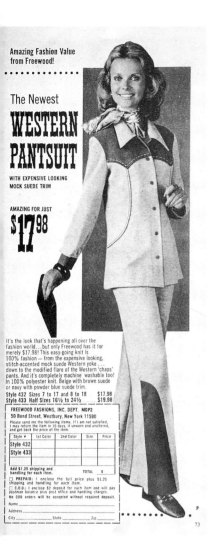

Advertisement for a polyester double-knit pantsuit, from *Photoplay*, February, 1977.

Polyester double-knit pantsuit with Mandarin collar, in a brown, blue, and white print. The bellbottom pants are hiphuggers.

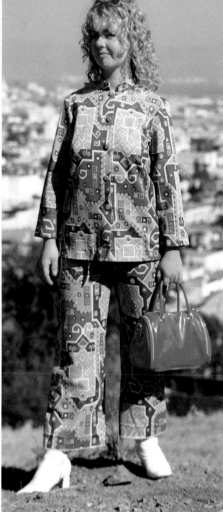

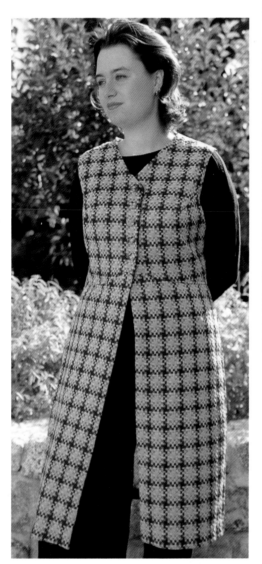

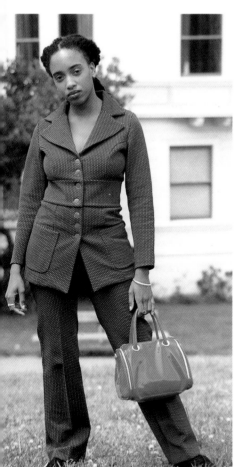

This long woven, lined vest originally went with matching wide-legged pants.

100% Dacron Polyester double-knit pantsuit has a wide, sewn-on belt that gives shape to the long, fitted jacket. It's royal blue with tiny pindots, and red buttons down the front of the jacket. The pants are bellbottoms.

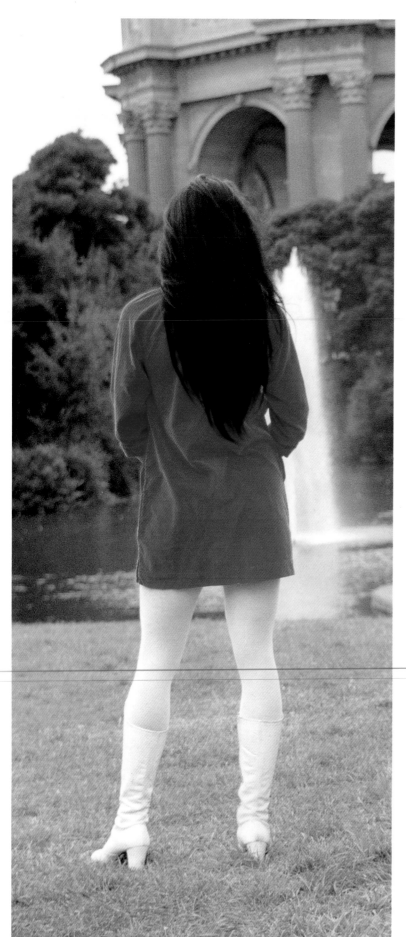

Bibliography

Calasibetta, Charlotte Mankey. *Essential Terms of Fashion: a collection of definitions*. New York: Fairchild Publications, 1986.

Calasibetta, Charlotte Mankey. *Fairchild's Dictionary of Fashion*. New York: Fairchild Publications, 1975.

Goldberg, Michael. *The Ties That Blind*. Atglen: Schiffer Publishing, Ltd., 1997.

Houck, Catherine. *The Fashion Encyclopedia: An Essential Guide to Everything You Need to Know About Clothes*. New York: St. Martin's Press, 1982.

Javna, John and Gordon. *'60s!*. New York: St. Martin's Press, 1983.

O'Hara, Georgina. *The Encyclopedia of Fashion*. New York: Harry N. Abrams, 1986.

Stegemeyer, Anne. *Who's Who in Fashion*. New York: Fairchild Publications, 1996.

Locations

The photographs in this book were taken in the following San Francisco locations: Noe-Beaver Pocket Park, Dolores Park, Mission Dolores, Alamo Square, the Haight-Ashbury, the Palace of Fine Arts, Duboce Park, my block and my backyard; and in Seoul, Korea.

Hot pink velveteen mini-dress. No label.

Value Guide

Fashions from the 1960s and '70s can still be found in a wide range of prices, depending on whether the item was discovered neatly pressed, on a hanger in a vintage shop, or dug from beneath a pile of old clothes at a flea market. In listing the values, I have decided to include both low-end and high-end prices. Of course there will be exceptions. I found the same pair of pop art bellbottoms selling in two different shops in two different cities, for $12.50 in one shop and for $200 in the other! Obviously, if I can get them for $12.50, even if I include the airfare to the other city, they're not worth $200 to me!

Clothes with designer labels, especially Pucci, go for much more than the values listed here. Pucci dresses can go for $125 - 275. If you can find one, like I did, for $8 at a garage sale, snap it up!

Bathing suits: $16 - 20
Bellbottoms: $12.50 - 16
Belts: $8.50 - 12.50
Boots: $12.50 - 40
Chain belts: $8.50 - 15
Cloth handbags: $8.50 - 15

Fabrics: $2 - 10
Fake fur: $16 - 55
Faux leopard: $50 - 100
Hats: $9.50 - 15
Hawaiian long dress: $14 - 20
Hawaiian short dress: $20 - 27
Hotpants: $9.50 - 12
Jumpsuits: $10 - 25
Leather handbags: $7 - 12.50
Leather jackets: $12.00 - $37
Long dresses: $10 - 35
Long skirts: $12.50 - 25
Maxi-coats: $24 - 38
Midi-coats: $12.50 - 28
Mini dresses: $8.50 - 30
Pantsuits: $15 - 25
Patchwork leather: $28 - 46
Patterns: $0.25 - 2
Plastic hats: $7 - 15
Plastic handbags: $7 - 60
Platforms: $28 - 40
Pleather jackets: $16 - 28
Scooter skirts: $13.50 - 15
Velvet jackets: $12.50 - 20

Index